Praise for
The Healthy Traveler

"*The Healthy Traveler* is fantastic — fun, practical, and medically accurate. From now on, I'm not leaving home without it. It's going to have a permanent home in my carry-on luggage."

Christiane Northrup, M.D.
Author of *The Wisdom of Menopause* and
  Women's Bodies, Women's Wisdom

"An entertaining little book packed with big ideas, full of proven remedies to prevent and relieve the stress and strain of travel. Tremendous. Take it along. You may wish you had if you don't!"

James Duke, Ph.D.
Author of *The Green Pharmacy*

"A treasure trove of good ideas and common sense for travelers who want to stay healthy while minimizing their use of pharmaceuticals."

Theresa Graedon, Ph.D.
Co-author of *The People's Pharmacy Guide to
  Home and Herbal Remedies*

"*The Healthy Traveler* is not only very informative and extremely useful, but also great fun to read. It provides quick remedies along with important preparation guidance to prevent the most common ills encountered when traveling. Highly recommended!"

Leslie Tierra, L.Ac., AHG
Author of *The Herbs of Life*
Co-founder, American Herbalists Guild

"This book should be available in every airport terminal, train or bus station, and seaport. Pack it in your bag. It offers valuable preventive measures and conventional, herbal, homeopathic, and other natural approaches."

Michael Tierra, OMD
Author of *The Way of Herbs*
Founder, American Herbalists Guild

"Highly recommended."

Luc Chaltin, N.D., D.I. Hom.
Founder, American Academy of Clinical
  Homeopathy
Author of *Homeopathy for First Aid and Common Ailments*

"I love this book! It's easy to read. It's funny. I love the summaries. You can read it for the fun of it or use it as a reference."

Frenesa Hall, M.D.

The HEALTHY TRAVELER

The HEALTHY TRAVELER

*A Handbook of Easy Solutions
for Common Travel Ailments*

Susan W. Kramer, Ph.D., AHG, Esq.

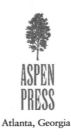

ASPEN
PRESS

Atlanta, Georgia

Published by Aspen Press, Atlanta, GA (aspen@earthways.com)
    For ordering information, visit
    www.earthways.com/healthytraveler

Edited and produced by Phyllis Mueller
Design and typesetting by Bonnie Supplee, Atlanta Georgia
Cover illustration by Marilyn King
Printing by Print Production Management
Author's photo by George Eckard
Travel vest by TravelSmith
The trademarks contained within are the property of their respec-tive owners.

Printed in the United States of America.
ISBN: 0-9713431-5-2

First Printing — October 2001

10 9 8 7 6 5 4 3 2 1

Dedication

To all my teachers

Acknowledgements

To my mother, Madeline Kramer, I am grateful for your gentle humor, your knowledge, and your acceptance of all my endeavors. To my late father, Eugene Kramer, "The Chief," an avid traveler who was always of service and who believed I could do anything, thank you.

Thanks to those who looked me straight in the eye and told me to start writing. To my teachers, Leslie and Michael Tierra of the East West School of Herbology, who advised me to begin book writing on the very first day we met and have continued encouraging me to this day, thank you.

Special thanks to Karen Tedeschi, DC, my healer, for unwavering friendship, wisdom, and support. Thanks to Charlene Hicks and Ronnie Entwhistle for guidance and encouragement. Thanks to my good friend Kim McCumbers of Heaven and Earth Consultations, who drove from Kentucky and devoted two weeks to the feng shui of my home to fully support me and my clients during the writing and production of this book.

For innumerable contributions, I am most grateful to Natalie Bravy, Wendi Dragonfire, Emmanuel Kaidanov, Alexandra Carrara, Linda McDowell, Esq., Andrew Reibman, Esq., Libby Eason Sener, Jan H. van der Veen, Ph.D., Martin Bronfenbrenner, Ph.D., Jill Ruttenberg, Patricia Kilpatrick, Sunny Mazur, AHG, Robyn Klein, AHG, Carol Hagen, Jenine Winborn, Marilyn Louise York, Wendy Papadenis, Jane Nelson, Farra Allen, Mark Blumenthal, AHG, Gael Carter, and Juaquita Callaway, MD.

To all of my clients, students, and workshop participants — it has been a privilege to work with you. Your experiences and feedback are woven into the fabric of this book.

To the listeners of *Health Talk with Susan Kramer* on WQXI-AM 790 in Atlanta, you consistently challenged me, taught me, and forced me to think outside the box. And yes, thank you for the show, where every caller asked, "When will you write your book and when does it come out?" Thanks to my producers, Bob Stamper, Robert Calhoun, and C.J. Faust, and my co-host, Dr. Ken Jackson, who took me by the hand, put me on the air, brought out my best, and repeatedly urged me to publish this material.

To my friend and editor, Phyllis Mueller, who shared my vision, produced this book, graciously accepted my lacunae, and provided unwavering support and technical expertise, my heartfelt thanks. To Bonnie Supplee, who created the wonderful design that perfectly matched my vision of this book, thank you. Thanks to Jane Bass for painstaking proofing. Thanks to Sonja Benjamin, Solange Bonnet, Tania Machado, and Mara Orlando — my language teachers — for the assistance with the Foreign Phrases.

To Leslie Tierra, L.Ac., AHG, Luc Chaltin, D.I. Hom., ND, Frenesca Hall, MD, and James Reinhardt, RP, many thanks for checking the content of and making contributions to this book. All of you generously gave your time, expertise, and encouragement. This book is better for your input.

Thanks to the students of the East West School of Herbology, the American Herbalists Guild, the Artists Conference Network, the Atlanta Women's Network, the National Women in Martial Arts Federation, Barbara Johnson's Open Door, the Atlanta Fencers' Club, The United States Fencing Association, and the Complementary and Alternative Medical Association (CAMA).

To Gary Zukav, Brugh Joy, Flenn Chrestman, Barbara Johnson, Anthony Robbins, and H.H. Tenzin Gyatso, the Fourteenth Dalai Lama, thank you and bless you.

Finally, I acknowledge all of you who read this book and use it to improve the quality of your life and travels. Thank you.

Susan W. Kramer
August 10, 2001
Atlanta, Georgia

Table of Contents

Introduction

I have always wanted a travel guide that would tell me what to do when emergencies arose. Preparing to dive the Great Barrier Reef and coughing up blood. Dealing with the inevitable constipation at conferences. Driving cross-country with a companion who became car sick on winding roads. At a remote country inn, my Dad running out of his needed water pill. A friend with food poisoning who was vomiting. Me with food poisoning and diarrhea. Arriving in Colorado Springs for the Olympic Trials and feeling the altitude. Hiking in the Rockies and experiencing altitude sickness. Difficulty falling asleep. Difficulty staying asleep. Tossing and turning all night. Feeling tired. I looked for over 30 years, but I've never found the guide I want. So I decided to write one, to provide the information a traveler is likely to need in one convenient, accessible place. Here it is.

I chose an easy-to-read format so you can find the information you are looking for without more stress. It is written in layperson's language with a minimum of medical jargon. It explains, step by step, how to deal with different problems. This handbook has the answers you need, emphasizing inexpensive and natural solutions and where to find them. It includes information on common travel ailments that can ruin a trip, ailments such as constipation, jet lag, stiffness, and blisters. I made it entertaining because I never liked those dry-as-dust medical books.

We have health problems when we travel that we rarely or never have at home. Because we don't have these problems at home, we don't think of them when we prepare to travel. This guide reminds you of common travel ailments so that you can plan ahead and assists you with travel solutions to problems you may not have anticipated.

Travel ailments can differ from at-home health problems because diet, clothing, schedule, and environment change with travel. We lose many of our anchors, many of our constants. Air travel exposes us to desert-dry air, decreased oxygen, and lower atmospheric pressure. Changing time zones upsets our internal clocks. We tend to do too much. We lift too much, talk too much, eat and drink too much. Increased quantities of food, salt, sugar, and fat, the hallmarks of most restaurant meals, all affect our digestion.

Travel involves change, and change is stressful. Increased levels of stress during travel increase the likelihood of illness. Stress exacerbates everything; many problems appear only under stress. People who never get sick fall ill. Athletes experience unexpected fatigue. Sound sleepers cannot fall asleep, and sometimes they cannot stay asleep. Normally relaxed people become tense and anxious. Eating while under increased stress plays havoc with digestion. Travel is stressful even under the best of circumstances, and not feeling your best makes it more stressful. The increased stress of travel creates many of the problems that you commonly experience during travel, but rarely experience otherwise.

The Healthy Traveler addresses travel ailments and their solutions. Major topics, such as constipation or jet lag, are organized into chapters. Chapters include personal experiences, specific instructions, food, herbal and drugstore remedies, and handy chapter summaries. When you need assistance with a travel problem, look first to the chapter headings. Alternatively, look up words relating to your problem in the index at the back of the book.

The remedies I selected for this book work well. They are drawn from western allopathic medicine, eastern and western herbalism, and homeopathy. The information in this book has been assembled from a variety of sources — personal experience, research of the medical and healthcare literature, advice and counsel of health professionals, and numerous case studies. Sometimes travelers know precisely what they need but that product (or healthcare tradition) may not be available for hundreds of miles — *The Healthy Traveler* assists you in finding effective substitutes. I firmly believe that "the herb you need grows in your own backyard." To paraphrase, you can find a solution close at hand, wherever you are in the world.

No matter how much I have learned over the years, when I am suffering, I find that all my education and knowledge disappears. My idea is that this travel guide will stay packed in your luggage, and that you'll find it so useful that you will remove it only to read when preparing for travel or for entertainment or information while traveling. It's meant to be handy. And it's affordable, so you can buy copies to give to friends who are planning trips. It is my hope that *The Healthy Traveler* addresses all your problems and answers all of your questions.

Happy, healthy traveling!

Susan

ALTITUDE SICKNESS

About 20 years ago, I qualified to compete at the U.S. Olympic Trials for fencing. I was thrilled! This was the first time I had qualified for the trials, and I was determined to do well. I had arrived in Colorado Springs and driven to the competition venue at the Air Force Academy. When I arrived at the gym, I took out my gear to begin practicing with my coach.

As I began pulling on my fencing jacket I noticed that my eyes were burning and I was having trouble focusing. I felt queasy. My head felt full, almost as if it were stuffed with cotton. My mouth was dry. I thought to myself, it must be nerves. I began lightly warming up, but my coordination was off. My coach called a halt, took off his mask, and told me to remove my gear.

A fencing master and jet fighter pilot from West Germany, my coach recognized the signs of altitude sickness. I wasn't the only person there who was feeling the effects. He instructed us to strip down to our running shorts, pull on our running shoes, and prepare for a cross country run. Explaining, he told us that we could suffer over the next few days or we could adjust to the new altitude more quickly. He advised the rapid method. We ran — gasping for air, our lungs burning, our guts twisting, and our heads pounding. I had never felt so sick on a run. Finally, we stopped. All of us collapsed on the ground. As I recovered my breath, my head was clear and I could focus. My headache was gone. Over the next few hours, my nausea completely passed.

We all had experienced altitude sickness. My home in Virginia was near sea level — the altitude at the venue was approximately 7,900 feet. I had rapidly moved from sea level to a height of approximately 1 1/2 miles, and this rapid ascent had created altitude sickness. Although it was mild and I could still function, my performance was impaired. I felt like a beginner, and I was not the only one. Many other competitors experienced nausea, headaches, and disorientation.

This was the first time that the Olympic Trials for fencing had been held in Colorado Springs. As I recall, the winner of the women's foil competition lived and trained at high altitude in Colorado. Fully adjusted to the altitude, she suffered no ill effects from it while most of her competitors did. (Talk about a home court advantage!) Although she was and still is an amazing athlete, she greatly exceeded expectations by winning. Me? I did my best, learned a lot, and watched the finals from the bleachers. (By the way, I do NOT recommend my coach's remedy.)

What Happens at High Altitude?

When altitude increases, air pressure decreases, resulting in less oxygen available for breathing. For example, at 8,000 feet the amount of oxygen drops to half the amount available at sea level. The decrease in oxygen means less oxygen reaches the blood. In response, people naturally begin to breathe more rapidly. Rapid breathing — in typically dry air — results in a loss of moisture.

When air pressure decreases, any pockets of air within the body increase in size, and may cause pain. Surgery often results in temporary pockets of air in the body that may persist for a week or more. If you recently have had surgery, even minor surgery, you may wish to delay activities involving rapid changes in air pressure, such as flying, climbing, or diving.

The increase in altitude also causes fluid in the blood to move into the body tissues, resulting in "thicker" blood and puffy wrists and ankles. You will retain water and may experience swelling in other areas of your body.

At higher altitude your risk of sunburn increases. At first, you may not notice the heat of the sun because the temperature tends to drop with increases in altitude. This can be even worse if you are climbing in snow or glacier areas where you will receive both direct and reflected sun rays. Even if clouds obstruct the sun, if it is daytime, those rays are coming through. When planning for high altitude, plan for protection against the blazing sun.

What Is Altitude Sickness?

Altitude sickness is the constellation of symptoms that result from experiencing high altitude or a rapid increase in altitude. These symptoms are related to the decrease of oxygen in the blood, the loss of moisture, and the slowing of waste elimination. Although not everyone will experience them all, symptoms include: Headache, nausea and vomiting, loss of appetite, insomnia, breathlessness, bleeding, coughing, anxiety or panic, inability to focus, disorientation, dizziness, and rapid heart rate.

The first signs of altitude sickness are decreased exercise performance and taking more breaths while at rest.

What Is High Altitude?

High altitude ranges from 4,950–11,500 feet (1,500–3,500 meters) above sea level.

Very high altitude ranges from 11,500–18,050 feet (3,500–5,500 meters) above sea level.

Extreme altitude includes all altitude above 18,050 feet (5,500 meters) above sea level.

How Bad Can Altitude Sickness Get?

You can die from altitude sickness. No joke.

Who Gets Altitude Sickness?

Anyone can get altitude sickness when he or she ascends to or stays at sufficiently high altitude. Mountain climbers. Trekkers. Automobile passengers. Visitors to ski resorts. Airline passengers (most jets are pressurized to the equivalent of an 8,000 foot altitude).

Travel communities that commonly deal with altitude sickness include trekkers in Peru, mountain climbers and trekkers in Nepal and the Himalayas, and visitors to Kathmandu.

Preventing Altitude Sickness

The best way to deal with altitude sickness is to avoid it. The medical mountaineering community has amassed considerable knowledge in this area. It is generally agreed that you cannot train for altitude except by experiencing altitude. (General physical conditioning may help.) Many recommend that you rest at an altitude at which you do not experience altitude sickness for at least 24–48 hours. If you are experiencing even mild symptoms, immediately descend. Descending even 500–1,000 feet may be sufficient to stop the symptoms.

When ascending above 8,000 feet, preferably

ALTITUDE SICKNESS

limit your ascent to 1,000–2,000 feet per day, with a 24 hour rest every 2–3 days. Yes, this is conservative. Mountaineers commonly recommend that you ascend 2,000–3,000 feet per day.

Let's say you are visiting Colorado Springs, which sits at approximately 8,000 feet. You've been there two days and you plan to climb Pike's Peak, which is approximately 14,000 feet. If you take the spectacular drive to the top, you can ascend 6,000 feet in about 1 hour. Most people who drive WILL experience varying degrees of altitude sickness (which will pass with time, medication, or simply descending). If you instead choose to climb Pike's Peak over a 2–3 day period, your prospects for altitude sickness sharply drop, and the severity of any symptoms also decreases. Over time, you adapt.

Both drinking at least 1–2 gallons of water per day and avoiding caffeine (found in coffee, tea, and chocolate) before and while ascending reduces the risk of altitude sickness. Interestingly, caffeine may alleviate symptoms once they begin. Alcohol seems to increase the risk. Tobacco seems to increase the risk.

Avoid highly salted foods, which are dehydrating.

Ascending and Descending

Taking your time greatly reduces the risk of

altitude sickness. Plan on taking at least two days to travel from sea level to 8,000 feet. After 8,000 feet, allow at least 1 day for each additional 2,000 feet of altitude. Schedule in a rest day for every 2–3 climbing days after reaching 8,000 feet.

Remedies for Altitude Sickness

Descend. Descending even 500–1,000 feet may eliminate all symptoms. Resting for a day, or even a few hours, at this level may be sufficient for your continued journey.

Drink more water. Dehydration is a symptom of altitude sickness and exacerbates it. At higher altitudes, dehydration occurs more rapidly. More rapid breathing speeds dehydration.

Oxygen helps. If you have access to oxygen, try it. Increased oxygen helps prevent and reduce the symptoms of altitude sickness. Depending upon the severity of symptoms, oxygen can eliminate coughing, revive flagging energy, and stop a headache. It can enable you to sleep at night. While it helps, oxygen might not be enough. Sometimes you've just got to descend and rest.

Homeopathic Remedies

Homeopaths recommend Coca 30c for the prevention and treatment of altitude sickness. (This is a specialty product; it will not get you high, and it does NOT contain cocaine!) Find homeopathic Coca on the Internet or contact a homeopath for further guidance.

Choosing Homeopathic Remedies

When shopping for homeopathic remedies, you will need to know both the name of the remedy and the potency. Obtaining the appropriate remedy is far more important than a particular potency. The potency is the number plus letter to the right of the remedy name on the label. I recommended 30c because that is the potency I use — it is generally available in my area, and it works well in first aid situations. If you cannot find 30c I recommend that you use potencies of 6x–30x or 6c–30c. A higher number indicates a higher potency.

Sometimes you may see homeopathic combination remedies for sale. Combination remedies are blends of several homeopathic medicines that address a group of related symptoms. They are generally labeled according to their use. If a single remedy is not available, or you can't decide which single remedy would be most appropriate, choose the combination remedy intended for your ailment.

Herbs

People have found a number of herbs helpful in dealing with altitude sickness.

Ginkgo leaf. I highly recommend ginkgo leaf to both prevent and treat altitude sickness. I like it because so many people find it effective, and it is extremely well tolerated. My physician friends like that they can find so much research, including at least one double blind study, demonstrating its value in preventing acute mountain sickness (AMS). (It also may help you to remember where you left your car keys.) As a preventative, I would take 1 dropperful of the tincture 3 times per day. As a treatment, I would take 1 dropperful every 1–2 hours, and I immediately would descend at least 500–1,000 feet.

Siberian ginseng. The next time that I travel to high altitude, I will use Siberian ginseng. This extensively researched herb increases aerobic capacity and endurance while increasing energy levels. The dose is 1 dropperful 3 times per day of the alcohol based tincture — you can take this dose hourly, as desired. I would use Siberian ginseng in combination with one of the other herbs in this section.

Reishi mushroom. You may find this under the names *ganoderma* or *ling zhi*. Like coca leaf (see below), it has a long history of traditional mountain use. Reishi is an Asian mushroom (although closely related species are found in the United States) that also is used to treat cancer and allergies and as an immune stimulant. It also is used to promote spiritual wisdom and is considered to be one of the most valuable herbs in the Chinese pharmacopoeia. Traditional Chinese medicine uses this herb specifically for asthma, coughing, insomnia, palpitations, dizziness, blood circulation, forgetfulness, and general debility. (Not surprisingly, those are many of the symptoms of altitude sickness.) The dose is 1 dropperful 3 times per day of the alcohol based tincture or 2 capsules 3 times per day to avoid altitude sickness. Take this dose hourly to treat altitude sickness.

Osha, a member of the *ligusticum* plant family, has been used traditionally by North American Indians for treating many respiratory problems, including pneumonia, bronchitis, asthma, and the common cold. They also used it to aid with breathing at high altitudes. While Indians chew a piece of the root to gain the benefits, you also can take osha tincture or capsules. The dose is 1 dropperful 3 times per day of the alcohol based tincture or 2 capsules 3 times per day to avoid altitude sickness. You can take this dose hourly to treat altitude sickness. Interestingly, osha typically grows at high altitudes.

Coca leaves. Yes, this is the source of cocaine and once was a key ingredient in Coca-Cola! Although possession or use of coca is prohibited in the United States, Canada, Great Britain, and other countries, you can legally possess and use it in Peru. Peruvian hotels serve coca tea. (Are you shocked? Cocaine is a highly refined product, but the plant's unrefined leaves are a mild stimulant, similar in effect to coffee or black tea.) Peruvian travel guides commonly give the leaves to trekkers to avoid and treat altitude sickness. Although coca has been used for centuries, trekkers report mixed success. (In my opinion, this may be because most trekkers travel according to a pre-set schedule that increases altitude too rapidly for them.)

Altitude Sickness Summary

Avoidance is best.
- Drink plenty of water.
- Avoid heavily salted foods.
- Avoid caffeine.
- Avoid alcohol.
- When climbing above 8,000 feet, allow 1 day for each 1,000–2,000 feet additional altitude, and rest for 24 hours every 2–3 days.

Treatment:
- Descend immediately at least 500–1,000 feet.
- Herbs:
  Ginkgo.
  Siberian ginseng.
  Osha.
  Reishi mushroom.
- Homeopathy:
  Coca 30c.
- Oxygen.

BITES

I had been hiking one day in the North Georgia mountains. It was one of those beautiful and perfect spring days. The dogwood trees were covered with white blossoms, and the hardwoods were filling out with fresh green leaves. The air was crisp, and you could smell the flowers.

I lay down, still breathing hard from the climb, on a grassy hill. I felt the sun warming my face and the cool dampness of the grass. I heard birds in the distance and my companions close by. I felt at peace.

Someone called my name and I turned my head. Suddenly, I felt a searing pain at my ear. The pain was so severe and so sudden that I had trouble seeing. I called to my companions. They didn't understand that something terrible had just happened, and they continued laughing and talking. The pain consumed me — I hurt so badly that I could not think. I felt helpless.

An elderly local man came and offered his assistance. As he helped me move into the shade and covered me with my jacket, he explained that I had been stung, probably by a bee. "A bee caused this kind of pain?" I asked. He told me that, depending where you are stung, the pain can be incredible. (It was!) He cautioned that although we would be able to numb the pain, it would continue for at least another 24–48 hours.

My new-found friend was right. We numbed the pain with a wad of chewing tobacco that we moistened with water and secured to my ear with a combination of Band-Aids and duct tape. The pain immediately decreased!

I was amazed at how quickly the tobacco worked. My ear still throbbed, but I could think again. When I touched the side of my face I could feel heat and swelling.

An ice pack pressed against my hot face provided temporary relief and gave me something to do. Aspirin helped slightly. When I removed the tobacco much of the severe pain returned so I quickly replaced my tobacco poultice. At home that night, I drank meadowsweet tea to reduce the pain and I slept with the tobacco poultice taped to my face. Towards the end of the second day the swelling and redness decreased. I awakened on the third day, pain-free.

Avoiding Bee and Other Insect Stings

Yellow jackets nest in dirt mounds, old logs, and dense shrubs. They also swarm at open food and open trash. When you're camping or picnicking, *cover your trash* and *don't leave food out*. Don't sit, eat, or rest near open trash or food. (Camp AWAY from the Dumpster.) While it may be difficult to avoid all of these, be aware when you are poking around! According to the Centers for Disease Control and Prevention, 70 percent of all insect stings are from yellow jackets. Each yellow jacket is capable of multiple stings, so watch out.

Honeybees nest in hives, work around flowers, and often light on the ground to forage for food. The majority of bee stings are to the soles of bare feet. *Wear shoes* to avoid being bitten on your feet and ankles from stepping on a bee. When a bee stings you, the stinger stays with you and continues pumping venom into you long after the bee leaves. Remove the stinger immediately. See "Treatment for Stinging Insects." When you are smelling the roses be aware of their other guests.

Hornets and wasps nest in a variety of places, including on and under roofs, under eaves, and on the sides of buildings. They may nest in hollow places such as walls and abandoned beehives or in trees or shrubs. A football-shaped papery object hanging from a tree branch likely is a hornet or wasp nest. *If you see a nest, leave it alone.*

Insects may be sharing your drink or food without your knowledge. When outdoors, LOOK each time you pick up your drink or take a bite. Open sugary drinks attract stinging insects, especially yellow jackets. Careful — one may have crawled inside your open can of soda.

If a stinging insect is near you, remain calm. DO NOT move quickly or aggressively; move slowly. If you swat or flail about, a stinging insect may interpret this as aggression and sting you. If the insect lights on you, breathe deeply and wait for it to leave. Be patient.

Talk calmly to any insect that is buzzing around you or has lit on you. (Shouting "get away"at the top of your lungs does not qualify.) Encourage the insect to leave by telling it where to go for food and create a mental image of that place. Say something simple like, "Please leave. Go to the flowers up the hill." Repeat your encouragement and directions until the insect leaves. This really works. (OK, so you think this is entirely stupid. Try it anyway. If nothing else, it reduces your anxiety level by giving you something to do. Eventually, the insect will leave without having stung you, and you will feel like Dr. Doolittle.)

Do not smash a stinging insect. If it is a yellow jacket, smashing it releases chemicals that alert fellow yellow jackets that war has been declared. DO NOT engage in warfare against stinging insects — you will lose.

Avoid looking or smelling like a flower! Bright colors and strong smells attract stinging insects. Entomologists tell us that yellow especially attracts, but that red does not. Flowery perfumes attract unwanted attention from stinging and biting insects — do not use them outdoors.

By the way, your insect repellent does NOT repel stinging insects! In fact, particularly smelly repellents may attract them.

Planning for Bee and Other Insect Stings

Stings from bees, wasps, hornets, and yellow jackets are unpleasant for everyone. At the least, you will experience a local response, which is restricted to the general location of the bite and may include pain that lasts for several days, skin irritation, swelling, and a welt. Some people additionally experience a systemic, or whole body, response. If it is not local, it is systemic. A systemic response may include red skin far from the bite, welts, general skin itching, nausea, and headache, all of which may arise within moments of the bite. A small percentage of people, about 2 percent, experience a severe systemic response, which may include eye, lip, tongue, and throat swelling, hoarseness, trouble breathing, dizziness, and fainting.

All stings require immediate treatment. Severe systemic response, also called anaphylactic shock (your throat closes up and you cannot breathe), requires immediate treatment plus medical attention.

You can die from a severe systemic response.

Most deaths from bites occur within one hour of the bite. Once you have experienced a severe systemic response you are at risk for the same or worse response the next time you are bitten.

If you have experienced a severe systemic reaction or anaphylactic shock from bee or other insect stings, consider it your responsibility to carry your own emergency aid. I recommend that you *carry a bee sting kit*, that you learn how to use it, and that you keep the kit readily available at all times — do not pack the kit at the bottom of your luggage! Do not rely upon your companions or even on local medical authorities for kits. Be prepared to take immediate action if you should get stung. If you cannot self-administer the kit, I recommend that you train someone in your group to assist you.

Kits include at least one, and preferably two or three, epinephrine pens (syringes), an antihistamine such as Benadryl, plus instructions. You can obtain epinephrine pens from your pharmacy with a doctor's prescription. While you are at the pharmacy, obtain an antihistamine. (Benadryl works very well but your doctor may recommend another drug or a stronger version of Benadryl.) The immediate use of an epinephrine pen plus an antihistamine can save your life, especially when medical care is far away. Ten helpful items for a bee sting kit are listed below.

Creating Your Bee Sting Kit

10 Helpful Items

1. Pen knife or expired credit card, for "flicking" stinger out.

2. 2–3 epinephrine pens (syringes): from pharmacy with doctor's prescription.

3. Antihistamine:
   Benadryl (diphenhydramine): from pharmacy, *and/or*
   Osha herbal tincture: from herb store or herbalist.

4. Homeopathic: Apis 30c, from health food store or homeopath. Made from bees, this is the most specific of remedies for bee sting. It also works well for other insect stings and for jellyfish stings. Taken immediately, it can stop anaphylactic shock. It specifically reduces swelling and the pain of the sting.

5. Antiseptic:
   2–3 alcohol wipes *or*
   Echinacea tincture *or*
   Tea tree oil or lavender essential oil.

6. 2–3 ice packs that cool when you break them

7. Topical pain killers:
   Lavender essential oil: apply every 15–30 minutes (also calming and relaxing) *or*
   Sting-Kill: from pharmacy.

8. Internal pain killer (optional):
   Herbal: 4 droppersful of meadowsweet or willow bark tincture, every 15 minutes.
   Pharmaceutical: Ibuprofen, aspirin, or acetaminophen.

9. Topical Antibiotic:
   Tea tree oil or lavender essential oil *or*
   Neosporin or other pharmaceutical antibiotic ointments.

10. Relaxant:
    Rescue Remedy flower essence *or*
    Chamomile herb tincture *or*
    Lavender essential oil.

BITES

Learn your options for treating insect stings and plan for them before you travel. Even a local response to a sting can ruin a trip. Carry a bee sting remedy with you.

Treatment for Insect Stings with Your Kit

Look for the stinger, which looks much like a tiny wooden splinter. If you see it, IMMEDIATELY *"flick" it out* with your fingernail, the edge of a knife, or a credit card. Do NOT pinch it out — you may force more venom into the skin! The stinger from some insects is a self-contained unit that continues pumping venom even though the insect has left. According to the CDC, even a five second delay can make a huge difference in the amount of venom that enters your system and the length of your recovery. Do NOT wait for the doctor.

If you know you are at risk of a severe systemic response, *use your epinephrine pen* NOW. Inject the syringe directly into your thigh. (You are at risk if you experienced a severe systemic response in the past and have not been de-sensitized to stings. Untreated, people become more sensitive over time.) Next, *take a dose of your antihistamine.* NOW call the doctor or begin travel to close-by medical attention.

If you are relying upon homeopathics and herbs, take your first dose of *Apis 30c* NOW and

BITES

repeat in 15 minutes or whenever you feel symptoms progressing. Take Apis by placing 1–2 pellets beneath your tongue and letting them slowly dissolve. While they are dissolving, swallow 2 droppersful or approximately 40 drops of *osha* herbal tincture. Repeat osha as needed to improve your breathing. Apis specifically neutralizes the effect of the insect toxin and osha acts as a natural antihistamine. Apis works for bee, wasp, hornet, and other insect stings and for a variety of other bites that create severe pain and possibly anaphylaxis. Divers and snorkelers stung by sea urchins or starfish additionally should take Silica 30c, dissolving 1–2 pellets beneath the tongue 3 times per day until symptoms cease. Homeopathic Silica assists your body in expelling the splinters and debris. Apis 30c, Ledum 30c, and Carbo veg. 30c are good choices for jellyfish stings. See "Choosing Homeopathic Remedies," page 12.

Wash the affected area with soap, water, and an antiseptic such as alcohol, tea tree oil, lavender essential oil, or echinacea tincture. This will reduce the risk of infection. You don't know where that stinger has been!

Apply ice directly to the sting site for 20 minutes to avoid and reduce swelling and to reduce pain. Continue to apply ice as needed. If the sting is to your leg or foot, elevate above the heart to reduce swelling and pain.

Topical pain-killers help. Apply 3–4 drops of *lavender essential oil* directly to the sting — lavender is a natural anodyne (pain-killer) and anti-spasmodic, and it will help you to relax. Re-apply every 15 minutes or whenever you feel the pain returning. Alternatively, look for *Sting-Kill* at your pharmacy. Sting-Kill contains benzocaine, which numbs the skin, and menthol, which reduces the itch. These remedies work surprisingly well!

The venom from flying stinging insects is what causes the itching and pain. Soak a cotton ball in *echinacea* tincture, tape it to the sting, and replace hourly — echinacea has strong anti-toxin qualities and will reduce the healing time. If you don't have echinacea, you can neutralize the alkaline venom by using a weak acid such as apple cider *vinegar*. *Baking soda*, which is weakly alkaline, is a good choice if you have neither echinacea nor vinegar. Many physicians will recommend cortisone or another steroid cream to reduce pain and itching.

Calm down. The more relaxed you are, the less pain you will feel! Breathe deeply. Take 4 drops of *Rescue Remedy* every 15 minutes. If you have lavender essential oil, put 1–3 drops on a cloth, bring it to your nose, and breathe deeply. Repeat as necessary. Alternatively, take a dropperful of chamomile tincture or a cup of strong chamomile tea every 30 minutes. Other helpful herbs include kava kava, passion flower, or valerian — take them the same as you would take chamomile but watch out — the valerian will make you sleepy.

Wilderness Treatment for Insect Stings

Follow the instructions above.

Neutralize the sting by applying "the best" remedy — *tobacco*. Take chewing tobacco, pipe tobacco, or open a cigarette — any tobacco will work — moisten with echinacea tincture, vinegar, water, or spit, and apply liberally to the sting. Tape or bandage this and change this dressing in 1–4 hours. Don't have tobacco? If you can locate it, *plantain leaf* works almost as well as tobacco. Pound the plantain leaf or rub it vigorously between your hands to break the cellular walls, moisten with echinacea tincture, vinegar, water, or spit, and apply the same as tobacco. Other alternatives include *wet mud, moistened clay,* or *moistened powdered charcoal.* Wet soil from a river or stream bed will work. The moistened mud, clay, or charcoal will draw out and neutralize the toxin. Apply the same way as tobacco.

Neutralize the alkaline venom of bees and wasps by applying your own spit directly to the sting — it is mildly acid. Did you bring any *aspirin* with you? Aspirin is acid — smash it to a powder, moisten, and apply to the sting. While you have the aspirin out, take 2 aspirins internally to reduce pain. If there are any willow trees close by, you can boil 2 tablespoons of the bark in 2 cups of water to make a tea to reduce your pain. Drink a half cup every 30 minutes. *Willow bark* contains salicylic acid, the primary ingredient in aspirin.

Apply ice or a cold pack if you have it. Using a cold compress — a cloth dipped in cold water — may ease discomfort.

Breathe! Pain decreases as your anxiety level decreases.

Desensitizing from Insect Stings

Anaphylactic shock is life-threatening, so it's no wonder the healthcare community has developed ways to desensitize susceptible individuals. Both allopathic physicians and homeopathic physicians use minute amounts of bees or bee venom to desensitize their patients. Allergists use allergy shots and homeopaths use oral preparations. Does desensitization work? For most people, yes.

People who experience anaphylactic shock from stings and who commonly are exposed to stinging insects can obtain desensitizing shots from their doctor. Allergists find the shots to be 90–95 percent effective at eliminating the anaphylactic response. Typically, you would receive shots 2 times per week for 10–20 weeks, and then taper down to 1 shot every 1–2 months for a period of 5 years.

Homeopathy offers a similar strategy. Consult a professional homeopath for personal guidance, and review one of the excellent texts on homeopathy for detailed descriptions of the underlying theory. To desensitize yourself, you would take 1 Apis 6x pill daily for 20–30 days. Cut back or stop if you begin experiencing any bee sting symptoms.

Planning for Insect Bites

I once took a summertime bike trip along the barrier islands of North Carolina. I had been told that the mosquitos were bad so I packed an insect repellent. We got out of our station wagon and into winds of 20 miles per hour. We unloaded the bikes, arranged our gear, and took off for Cape Hatteras. We rode peacefully for an hour, noticed that the wind had died down, and stopped to rest. Arrgh! There must have been thousands of mosquitos! Where had they come from? Our shorts and tank tops provided no protection. My friend must have had a hundred mosquitos just on one arm. They were in our eyes and we madly swatted at them. We jumped and yelled and scrambled to pull cans of spray repellent from the bikes. We took turns spraying each other and gradually began to breathe again.

Later, we learned that mosquitos in that area

peak in late summer to early fall. Had we arrived in the spring, we might not have encountered any mosquitos. At the next store, we purchased additional repellent — just in case.

Avoiding Mosquito and Other Insect Bites

During the warm months in many parts of the world, biting insects are a fact of life. Mosquitos, gnats, biting flies, fleas, and ticks are common pests. If you will spend time outdoors, plan for bites.

Cover up. Long-sleeve shirts with cuffs, long pants with elastic cuffs, socks, and hats provide protection.

Avoid wearing blue. The color blue attracts mosquitos.

Chemical insect repellents work. Repellents containing DEET are very effective but may also be the most toxic. If you use them, especially on children, spray the clothes and not the skin. Do NOT spray pets with DEET. Remember, with pets and with small children, what goes on the pet or child goes in the pet or child. Wash your hands after using DEET.

Natural insect repellents work. Available at health food stores and outdoors stores, these typically contain essential oils such as citronella and lemongrass. Many are pleasant smelling and do not present the toxicity problems of chemical repellents.

They are a great choice especially in low to medium infestation areas.

Eat lots of garlic. When you eat garlic, your skin exudes "eau de garlic." Mosquitos don't like the smell. (Unfortunately, your companions may not appreciate it either!)

Don't eat sugar and cut back on fruits and fruit juices. Yes, eating sweets makes you smell sweet, especially to mosquitos. Perfume, scented deodorants, and after-shave also may increase your attractiveness to mosquitos.

Try a solar powered "mosquito guard." This device, which you wear on your belt or put in a pocket, emits a barely audible whine that discourages mosquitos. It's inexpensive and available from mail order catalogues. I have a mosquito-sensitive friend who swears by hers.

Treating Insect Bites

- Immediate washing with soap and water will eliminate symptoms of many bites.
- Homeopathic Apis 30c or Ledum 30c will eliminate symptoms for many people. The dose is 1 pill every 15 minutes until the symptoms cease or moderate. The earlier you do this, the more effective the remedy. Arnica 30c, if you do not have Apis or Ledum, will reduce swelling.
- Lavender essential oil, applied directly to the bite,

will reduce pain and swelling. The dose is 1–3 drops. This works for a wide range of bites, including mosquito and spider bites. Tea tree oil is a good second choice. Re-apply whenever the pain or itching returns.

- Chickweed is one of the best herbal remedies for itching. You can find it growing wild in many temperate areas (especially in the lawn, at curbs, and at the sides of buildings). It also is widely available at health food stores. Pound and moisten fresh chickweed or moisten dry chickweed, apply and tape to the bite, and replace every few hours. If you don't see any chickweed, plantain works almost as well. Or use one of the many excellent herbal salves containing chickweed.

- Ammonia or apple cider vinegar, applied directly to the bite, takes the sting and itch out of many bites. If one doesn't work, try the other. Ammonia works especially well on mosquito bites. (Some drugstore products use ammonia as the active ingredient to eliminate mosquito bite itch.)

- Baking soda mixed with water takes the sting out of many bites and is especially helpful with ant bites.

- Cortisone or other steroid creams relieve itch. Benadryl cream relieves itch.

- If bites result in a systemic response — that is, if your breathing becomes impaired or you develop red patches where you haven't been bitten — take internally an antihistamine such as osha herbal tincture or Benadryl. Seek medical attention for impaired breathing.

BITES

Bites Summary of Remedies

Avoid getting bitten:
- Be aware. Avoid nests.
- Cover food and drink. Wear shoes.
- Remain calm. Move slowly. Do not swat or kill.
- Avoid bright colors (esp. yellow, blue), strong smells.

Plan for stings and bites:
- Act quickly.
- If allergic, carry an epinephrine pen (prescription only).
- Create a sting and bite kit — keep it handy.

Treatment of insect stings and bites:
- Remove stinger.
- Western medicine: Use epinephrine pen, take antihistamine.
- Holistic: Take homeopathic Apis 30c, osha root tincture.
- Wash. Apply antiseptic (alcohol, tea tree oil, echinacea tincture).
- Ice. Elevate.
- Pain and itch reduction: Lavender oil or Sting-Kill. (Or use vinegar, ammonia, baking soda, or a steroid cream.)
- Calm down: Breathe. Rescue Remedy. Lavender oil. Chammomile.

Wilderness treatment of insect stings:
- Tobacco. Mud, moistened clay, charcoal, spit, aspirin, willow bark, or plantain leaf.

Desensitizing treatments:
- Allergy shots.
- Homeopathy. Apis 6x pills.

Avoid mosquito and other bites:
- Cover up. Wear shoes and socks.
- Chemical and natural repellents. CAUTION: DEET.
- Eat garlic. Avoid sweets.

Treatment of mosquito and other insect bites:
- Wash with soap and water.
- Homeopathy: Apis 30c, Ledum 30c, or Arnica 30c.
- Essential oils: Lavender or tea tree.
- Herbs: Chickweed or plantain.
- Kitchen remedies: Ammonia, vinegar, or baking soda.
- Pharmaceutical remedies: Cortisone cream or Benadryl.

BLEEDING

Ten years ago I was in Cairns, Australia taking a deep sea diving course so I could dive the Great Barrier Reef. Wow! I already had tickets for the dive boat and was planning to spend a week diving. On the third and final day of the dive course, as I was walking to the dive school, I cleared my throat and tasted blood. BLOOD? I never spit up blood! I was experiencing minor hemorrhaging from the water pressure. What could I do? If I continued to bleed, I would be DQ'd, disqualified, from diving.

I went searching for an herb to stop the bleeding. I looked first for comfrey, which grows wild. I knew comfrey to be one of the best anti-hemorrhaging agents — it would stop the bleeding fast. I was confident in my choice, but could not find the herb, either in the field or in the local herb shop. I also looked for cattails. Cattails, which grow in abundance in so many places, are great remedies for bleeding. Alas, they were not available.

Not knowing what else to do, I told my instructor who sent me to the school doctor. I asked, "Isn't there something [a drug] you can give me to stop the bleeding?" I thought to myself, this had to be a very common problem. The doctor shook his head. No.

He pulled a paper from the stack on his desk, signed it, and handed it to me. The doctor had disqualified me. I could snorkel; I could not dive. Without the high water pressure from diving, my bleeding gradually stopped on its own. (I did go out on the dive boat and enjoyed snorkeling. The Great Barrier Reef really is worth the trip.)

Years later, I was struck in the face by the hatch on a minivan. The hatch suddenly had flown upward, embedding my wire-rimmed glasses a quarter inch into the bridge of my nose. Blood streamed down my face. I removed the glasses, and the blood flowed faster. I washed the wound with soap and water, hoping the soap would stop the bleeding. It did not. The blood continued to flow.

This time I was prepared. I pulled a jar of a *comfrey-based salve* from my purse and pressed some into the cleaned wound. The bleeding stopped within 30 seconds! I stood looking at myself in the restroom mirror. Blood began seeping from my wound, I smeared on more salve and the bleeding ended. Despite the depth of the cut, my wound healed rapidly and without a scar.

Although a styptic pencil will stop bleeding from small cuts (ever watch boxing?), I know of no drug that stops bleeding. To stop bleeding from large cuts or wounds, western medicine relies on pressure and surgery.

Basic First Aid for Bleeding

When dealing with a bleeding cut, *applying firm pressure* to the wound, preferably with a clean cloth such as a T shirt or scarf, may stop the bleeding. *Wash* the wound thoroughly with soap and water. This initial washing is critical, especially for puncture wounds, to reduce the risk of infection. Remember the old Western movies, where the doctor liberally poured whiskey into the wound? The whiskey served a double purpose: cleaning the wound and killing bacteria in it.

Herbal First Aid for Bleeding

Herbs give you an additional tool to stop external and internal bleeding beyond the application of direct pressure. Hemostatic herbs (herbs that will stop bleeding) are widely available. *Shepherd's purse*, a common weed that I've seen growing at roadsides, at the edges of trails, in horse pastures, and at the edges of grassy fields, will stop internal and external bleeding. (It works well at reducing women's bleeding between cycles.) Although the fresh plant is considered superior to the dried, even the dried will work in a pinch. Tinctures made from the fresh plant, available in health food stores, seem to work best. Take 1– 4 droppersful hourly until the bleeding stops.

I usually combine shepherd's purse with *yarrow*.

Yarrow is my all-time favorite remedy to stop nose-bleeds. Yarrow grows wild and is gaining populari-ty as a garden flower. Again, I recommend a tinc-ture, given in the same dosage as shepherd's purse. Both the dried and fresh yarrow work well. Yarrow can be prepared as a tea: Add 2 tablespoons of the dried flowers and leaves to 1 cup recently boiled water and let steep for 10–20 minutes.

You can stop external bleeding by applying a hemostatic (stop bleeding) herbal tincture or salve directly to the wound — comfrey, yarrow, shep-herd's purse, and tienchi ginseng all work well. Sprinkling *cayenne pepper* directly on the wound and holding it closed works well — alternatively, you could apply a poultice consisting of moistened fresh or dry herb to the wound. Poultices are easy to prepare and very effective.

Preparing a Poultice

To prepare a poultice, grind, rub, or pound 1–4 table-spoons of herb (to break the cell walls), moisten with tincture, tea, or pure water, place on plastic wrap or some other non-porous surface (even a Band-Aid), and apply directly to the wound. Secure in place with tape, a towel, a scarf, an elastic bandage, or what-ever you have.

My favorite remedy to stop bleeding is *comfrey*. The botanical name is *Symphytum officinale*. It will stop hemorrhaging anywhere in the body (although I haven't tried it for uterine bleeding) and works well with both internal and external bleeding. Comfrey taken internally will stop lung bleeding (coughing up blood), stomach bleeding (usually seen as black stool), and colon bleeding. Of course, you should see a healthcare provider for any of these conditions.

Comfrey in any form will work. Fresh or dried, leaf or root. It grows wild in many areas and is available in many health food stores in the United States and on the Internet. If it is unavailable in stores where you live and you do not have access to the Web, I suggest that you grow your own. I think everyone should have a comfrey plant. It is easy to grow, quite hardy once it becomes established, and easily propagated from a piece of the root. (Be aware that comfrey can become invasive and dominate its area of the garden. Also, comfrey is very tenacious — choose your location wisely because it will "insist" on returning even if you dig it up.)

Caution: Comfrey, when used externally, can work too well! Not only will it stop the bleeding, but it will cause the tissue it touches immediately to begin healing. Really immediately. That means that you MUST thoroughly clean any wound prior to applying comfrey or you risk a nasty infection. It also means that you should NOT apply comfrey to a puncture wound — you run a major risk of abscess.

THE SAFE USE OF COMFREY

I and others consider comfrey an invaluable remedy that has been used safely for centuries by millions of people. Some authors criticize the internal use of comfrey due to the possible presence of pyrrolizidine alkaloids (PAs). If you choose to use comfrey and also choose to avoid the pyrrolizidine alkaloids: (a) only use comfrey which has the botanical name, *Symphytum officinale*: this species has lower PAs than other species and is the species that commonly grows in the United States; (b) only use comfrey leaf: the leaf has much lower PA levels than the root; and (c) consider using "pyrrolizidine free" comfrey preparations. *The Botanical Safety Handbook* by the American Herbal Products Association recommends that you limit (daily) internal consumption to 4 to 6 weeks per year and that you substitute other herbs if you have liver problems, are nursing, or are pregnant.

People use comfrey salves to speed healing for a wide variety of ailments. Do NOT use the salves on deep or puncture wounds unless those wounds have been thoroughly irrigated and cleaned. Comfrey works amazingly fast; the tissue that it touches first will heal first and debris trapped in a deep wound could cause infection. *The Botanical Safety Handbook* does not caution about PA content for the salves but advises that nursing mothers use other remedies for breast tenderness.

Why do I rate comfrey so highly? It is cheap, I've never seen a negative effect, and it works. It also will accelerate healing from any injury and from overexertion. It is my favorite post-surgical remedy. Formerly called "knitbone," it will greatly speed healing of (properly set!) broken bones. It will speed the mending of cracked ribs or a sprained ankle.

Chinese herbalists and an increasing number of western herbalists and naturopathic doctors favor *Yunnan Paiyao* to stop internal and external bleeding. Yunnan Paiyao is a Chinese "patent medicine" — a commercially available combination of herbs. The formulation has been kept secret for many years, although we know that the main ingredient is *tienchi ginseng*. (Tienchi ginseng also will stop bleeding.) It comes in an orange pill or powder contained within a small vial, topped by a tiny red pill.

Yunnan Paiyao may be taken internally (up to 3–4 doses per day) and the powder may be sprinkled directly on the wound. (I personally avoid placing anything in a wound, other than soap, water, or alcohol, unless the bleeding will not stop.) What about the tiny red pill? The pill is taken only for severe hemorrhaging, and is commonly used in the East by police for gunshot wounds. Yunnan Paiyao is inexpensive, easy to pack, and can be found in Oriental markets and Chinese herb shops.

Cayenne pepper will stop bleeding, both internally and externally. Not as powerful as comfrey or tienchi ginseng, it is readily available from a

BLEEDING

kitchen, grocery store, or restaurant. For use on cuts, sprinkle directly into the cut, hold the edges of the cut closed for 2–5 minutes, and breathe calmly as you wait for the bleeding to stop. Interestingly, most people find that it does not sting on a simple cut (but it will sting on a scrape). Mixing a teaspoon of cayenne into a half cup of water and drinking it will slow and even stop bleeding. It also will warm you! Uncooked, it will not create the burn you experience with spicy foods. This is one of the very best kitchen remedies and is easy to carry in capsules.

Speaking of kitchen remedies, if nothing else is available, try *vinegar*. Take a quarter teaspoon vinegar every fifteen minutes until the bleeding stops. I think of vinegar as a great emergency remedy for nosebleed or spitting up blood. You can find vinegar in kitchens, restaurants, and food stores around the world.

When all else fails or if nothing else is at hand, use *ashes*. Ashes? Yes. Ashes are one of the BEST ways to stop external bleeding. The Chinese traditionally use the ash from moxa — which is made from mugwort — by sprinkling it into the wound. You can use ashes from burnt wood or even from burning your own hair! Why is this remedy listed last? Because it WILL cause tattooing (skin discoloration) that will persist for some time.

Bleeding in the Wilderness

As a child, I wanted to know what plant or what tree you could use to stop bleeding. What if my friends and I were stuck in the woods (which were adjacent to our backyard) and Johnny fell, struck his head on a sharp stone, and began bleeding to death? What would we DO? (Home was only 50 yards away, but what if?)

I decided to learn which plants stop bleeding. The *Junior Girl Scout Handbook* was no help; the *Boy Scout Handbook* also had no information on hemostatic (stop bleeding) herbs. I asked every adult who I thought should know what I thought was basic and life-saving information. I asked medical doctors, nurses, and veterinarians. None of them knew.

Over the years, I learned that some people did know. I met naturalists, park rangers, and Native Americans who knew emergency wilderness medicine and knew how to use plants to stop bleeding. I was surprised to learn that many herbs that stop bleeding are easily identified shrubs and trees. Later, I found extensive documentation supporting this use of plants, and I saw plants stop bleeding. I highly recommend that wilderness hikers learn to identify at least a few of the plants that stop bleeding. As an added bonus, most of these plants also stop diarrhea! (Obtain a good field guide that

B L E E D I N G

illustrates and describes medicinal plants in your area. Depending where I am, I hike with *A Field Guide to Medicinal Plants and Herbs of Eastern and Central North America* (Peterson Field Guides) by Steven Foster and James A. Duke or *Medicinal Plants of the Mountain West* by Michael Moore. You can find field guides for most areas of the world.)

Cattail pollen, from the brown fuzzy spike that grows along roadsides, in swamps, and alongside streams and ponds, is an excellent remedy to stop both internal and external bleeding. To use, shake the brown and fuzzy part in a bag or cloth and collect the yellow pollen. Place the pollen on the bleeding area. Bleeding will immediately slow. For severe hemorrhaging, mound up the pollen on the cut and secure with a bandage or clean cloth. Stirring a teaspoon of the pollen into water and drinking it will reduce bleeding from the inside. Roasting the pollen first will increase the potency. Roast it by heating in a dry skillet until the pollen begins to brown, and then remove from heat. I especially like cattail pollen as a wilderness remedy because it is so easily identified. The ONLY drawbacks to cattail pollen are that the pollen is available only in late spring or early summer, and many states in the United States prohibit gathering it. (It DID grow in the woods behind our house.)

Comfrey, mentioned above, is an outstanding remedy to stop bleeding. Simply pressing the leaves on the wound will stop bleeding. Bruising the leaves by pounding or rubbing them will increase the effectiveness. Can't find any? Try to find one of the other remedies on this list.

Yarrow, a common garden and wildflower, is another great choice. I would use the leaves. Bruise the leaves and press directly on the wound. A tea made from a quarter cup of the flowers and leaves simmered for 10–20 minutes in a cup of water will slow both internal and external bleeding. It also slows diarrhea. (It is one of my favorite remedies. When you begin coming down with a cold, try sipping a half cup of the tea every hour.)

Plantain is a very common roadside and trailside plant that grows prolifically throughout temperate regions. It's nicknamed "white man's foot" because it is most commonly found in high traffic and disturbed areas. Both the narrow (lance leaf) and round (broad leaf) varieties slow bleeding. Use the leaf to slow bleeding and also to fight infection. Used externally, the crushed fresh leaf kills bacteria and slows bleeding. Use it to heal trauma, open sores, and bleeding wounds. Taken internally as a tea, it helps to fight infection and even will help to clear urinary tract infections.

The leaf and root of *wild blackberry*, *wild*

raspberry, and *wild strawberry* plants all slow bleeding and diarrhea. The root is stronger than the leaf; use the root to make tea while pressing the well-bruised leaf against the wound. The leaf tea is also a tasty beverage. Simmer a quarter cup of leaf in 2 cups of water for 20–30 minutes and drink a half cup every 15–30 minutes.

Having trouble recognizing the small plants? The mighty *oak* tree — easy to recognize by its acorns — helps to stop bleeding. Although it may not work as quickly as cattail, comfrey, or yarrow — it will work. Prune a small branch, strip off the outer bark, and use the inner bark. Make a poultice to stop external bleeding, or simmer 2 tablespoons of the bark in 2 cups of water for 20 minutes and sip to stop internal bleeding or diarrhea. Can't wait? Use the leaves to make a poultice while waiting for the bark preparation. The white oak is considered the best of the oaks therapeutically, but I will happily use any oak I find.

In an emergency, if I could find nothing else, I would confidently use clean *campfire ashes* or *ashes from burned human hair*. I would accept the temporary tattooing in return for saving a life.

Bleeding Summary of Remedies

Top choices of "packable" bleeding remedies (you only need one):

- Comfrey tincture or capsules.
- Yunnan Paiyao vials.
- Shepherd's purse tincture.

Other excellent choices:

- Yarrow tincture.
- Cayenne capsules.
- Tienchi ginseng tincture, powder, or capsules.

Kitchen remedy:

- Vinegar.

Top choices for wilderness remedies:

- Cattail pollen.
- Comfrey leaf.
- Yarrow leaf.
- Blackberry, raspberry, and strawberry leaf and root.
- Plantain leaf.
- White oak inner bark.
- Ashes.

BLEEDING

BLISTERS

As a traveler, martial artist, and athlete, I have had my share of blisters. There are so many blister stories to tell! Still, one stands out.

My roommate and I were new students at Marlboro College in Vermont. We were looking forward to the weekend — she would travel to Bear Mountain for a hiking trip and I planned to participate in on-campus activities. On Friday afternoon she walked into our room, exuberant, carrying a large box. We plopped on her bed. She opened the box and pulled out a brand new pair of heavy duty all-leather Dunham hiking boots. They were great! We admired them. They were the ultimate in style for a school obsessed with the outdoors.

My roommate had a choice: She could wear her old, ratty, stained, scuffed, and comfortable boots or she could wear her brand new all-leather Dunham hiking boots with the trendy Vibram lug soles. It did not take long to decide. After all, this was to be a short hike. She was going to climb Bear Mountain, camp at the top, and climb down the next day. She knew that hiking boots required a breaking-in period; she decided to break them in on the hike.

My roommate wasn't looking for advice.

On Saturday she pulled on heavy hiking socks

but had trouble lacing her boots, so she changed to a thin pair of socks that also matched her shorts. These socks were dirty, so she quickly washed them and dried them as well as she could by rolling them in a towel. "I'll be fine," she said as she ran for the waiting car.

She looked great.

The hike was longer and more challenging than anyone had imagined, and I heard those socks stayed wet all the way to the top of Bear Mountain. (Did I forget to say it was freezing and that no one had planned for cold?) My roommate reported that her feet ached on the way up. The boots pinched in some places, rubbed in others, and generally felt hard. But walking up was nothing compared to walking down. Her feet burned all the way. She felt her feet sliding forward in her boots. She feared she was shredding her feet but was too embarrassed to complain or ask for help.

My roommate limped into our dorm room on Sunday night. We closed the door, and I helped her to her bed. Gingerly, I helped pull off her boots and peeled off her socks. What a sight! Her feet were damp, wrinkled, and scattered with Band-Aids. Some Band-Aids appeared to have shifted, judging from the gray glue residue on much of her skin. Many spots were red. The top layer of skin had begun separating from her feet, the skin filled with

BLISTERS

fluid. Blisters had formed. Blisters beneath Band-Aids were intact, but most of the other blisters had torn. We gently washed her feet and sprayed them with Bactine. She wore sandals for the next few days. I became interested in blisters.

Those of us who wear brand new shoes for long journeys ought to plan for blisters. Blisters happen. They also happen to folks who DO break in their footgear but are not accustomed to the intensity of their journeys.

What Are Hot Spots and Blisters?

Hot spots are painful, red areas on the skin surface that have been caused by friction. If the friction continues, hot spots become blisters.

Blisters are raised, fluid-filled bubbles of skin. Blisters typically are caused by friction or by intense or prolonged heat. They actually are a separation of the layers of skin. Blisters may be filled with blood, in which case they are called blood blisters or hematomas. Blisters may be small or large. Blisters easily may range from 1 centimeter in diameter to large (50 centimeter) coin-sized blisters that cover the feet (or any other exposed skin).

Blisters can ruin an otherwise wonderful trip. They can be surprisingly painful and may engage all of your attention. Blisters may physically prevent you from wearing certain shoes because of swelling,

BLISTERS

bleeding, oozing, or pain. Blisters can stop you from sightseeing, trekking, or even going to dinner. Infection may additionally complicate blisters.

Avoiding Hot Spots and Blisters

To avoid hot spots and blisters, *stay dry* and *reduce chafing*. As a general rule, *get a good fit* with all of your gear. Anything that rubs against your body for a long enough period of time will cause hot spots and blisters. *Talcum powder* and *cornstarch* absorb moisture and reduce chafing — and *powdered slippery elm bark* or *marshmallow root* provide additional relief. (Caution: Do not inhale talcum powder and do not use near bodily orifices — internal exposure to talcum powder increases the risk of cancer.) Many athletes use *tape* or *moleskin* directly on the skin where they know friction occurs. Athletes commonly tape their feet and hands. *Specialty fabrics* (such as CoolMax) that wick moisture away from the skin will keep you drier than most other fabrics.

For walkers, hikers, and runners, wearing good-fitting shoes is a must. Too tight or too loose WILL result in hot spots and blisters. DON'T purchase shoes that are a half size too large or too small just because they are on sale. For long hikes and treks, plan on wearing two pairs of socks — a thin inner pair (silk is a good choice) and a thicker outer pair

BLISTERS

to reduce friction. When you purchase your hiking and trekking boots, size them while wearing both pairs of socks. Many specialty shops and mail-order providers sell silk socks and glove liners. Many trekkers prefer single socks with double-layer soles.

Cyclists, you need to take the time to find gloves, shoes, and a seat that fits YOUR body. Blisters around the groin and buttocks are no laughing matter — and they are common. Many cyclists wear padded cycling pants or cycling pants with a chamois or synthetic chamois crotch — these reduce friction and provide an extra layer between you and the bike. Again, powder and cornstarch are very helpful; apply either one liberally. (Ladies, no talcum powder here, please!) If your hands blister, even with gloves, consider padded handlebar tape. Also, have you and your bike checked for proper fit. A few minor adjustments to your bike could increase your comfort level.

For travelers carrying or dragging bags, adjust all straps to provide the best fit for you. If the straps or handles still cut into or rub against you, consider padding them to make them softer or buy replacement straps from a luggage shop. Also, consider strengthening or reinforcing your skin with additional clothing, Band-Aids, or tape. Wear gloves.

Travelers may "toughen" feet and hands prone to blisters by soaking them in cold *black tea* or by

BLISTERS

applying black tea bags. The tannins in the tea strengthen the skin and reduce the likelihood of blisters.

Use *soap* to reduce friction on potential hot spots. Spread 2–3 drops of water on a bar of soap (bar soap works much better than liquid soap for this purpose) and rub the moistened soap over all high friction areas. This remedy especially helps you to adjust to increased activity levels. Use soap alone or in combination with moleskin.

Treating Hot Spots and Blisters

Treat hot spots or blisters immediately. Quick action may enable you to avoid a blister or eliminate one that has already begun. Even tough guys get blisters — treating yours immediately will save you time and discomfort down the road.

Soothing herbal salves and oils speed recovery from hot spots. A single drop of *lavender essential oil*, rubbed into a hot spot, may eliminate it by morning. Other excellent herbal solutions include *St. John's Wort* oil, salve, or tincture; *calendula* oil, salve, or tincture; or *comfrey* oil, salve, or tincture. When possible, leave the hot spot uncovered and exposed to the air until you are ready to resume your activity.

When you are ready to resume your activity, cover any hot spots. A simple Band-Aid may be suf-

BLISTERS

ficient. First aid tape works well. (Even duct tape works when you have no other tape available.) *Self-adhesive moleskin* is an excellent choice. If the hot spot is small, cut a hole in the center of some moleskin a little larger than the hot spot and position over the hot spot. Alternatively, place some cotton or gauze over the hot spot and cover with a larger piece of mole skin. Tough Skin, a liquid preparation that dries on contact, provides an additional layer of "skin." It does work, although debates continue as to whether it is superior to these other methods. A new product called Second Skin is positioned directly over the hot spot and taped into place. Some wilderness medicine physicians recommend it.

Blisters present more difficulties than hot spots. Apply a drop of *lavender essential oil* directly to the blister. This will reduce any pain, reduce the likelihood of infection, and accelerate healing. Tearing or puncturing a blister increases the risk of infection, so avoid this when possible. If you must puncture a blister, for example, if a blister is large, painful, and prevents necessary walking, do what you can to reduce the risk of infection.

To puncture and dress a blister:
1. Gently wash the blistered area with soap and clean water. Pat or air dry.
2. Sterilize a needle or tip of a knife by holding it in

BLISTERS

a flame. Wipe the needle or knife clean on a cloth
moistened with alcohol.

3. Pierce the edge of the blister, inserting the needle
   or knife tip just far enough to express fluid from
   the blister.

4. Gently press the blister to release the fluid.

5. Apply a drop of lavender essential oil, tea tree oil,
   iodine, echinacea tincture, alcohol, or antibiotic
   directly to the opening.

6. Position Second Skin or another commercial
   dressing directly over the blister and tape into
   place. Alternatively, use a Band-Aid.

To continue treating a blister:

1. Additional tape will reduce friction. Be sure to
   eliminate all wrinkles in the tape and bandage.
   The wrinkles also create blisters.

2. When possible, change the dressing daily and re-
   apply an essential oil (tea tree or lavender), echinacea tincture, or antibiotic ointment.

3. When possible, air dry the blistered area daily,
   preferably for four or more hours. If the blister is
   torn, apply an essential oil (tea tree or lavender)
   or echinacea tincture, and coat the skin with a
   comfrey herbal salve or an antibiotic ointment.

BLISTERS

Blisters Summary of Remedies

Avoid blisters:

- Keep high friction areas dry.
- Good fitting shoes and gear.
- Powder to absorb moisture and reduce chafing:
  Talcum *or* cornstarch *and*
  Slippery elm bark *or* marshmallow root.
- Moleskin or tape.
- Soap.
- Wear 2 pairs of socks.

Treating hot spots and blisters:

- Immediate treatment — do not delay.
- Herbal salves and oils speed recovery:
  Lavender essential oil *or*
  St. John's Wort, calendula, or comfrey oil, salve, or
  tincture.
- Expose to air when resting, cover when active.
  Band-Aid, first aid tape, moleskin, Tough Skin, or
  Second Skin.
- Apply an antiseptic to open blisters:
  Lavender essential oil or tea tree oil *or*
  Echinacea tincture *or*
  Iodine or alcohol *or*
  Antibiotic ointment.
- Change the dressing on open blisters daily.

BLISTERS

CONSTIPATION

Many of us get constipated when we travel. Why? Nerves, inactivity, lack of fluids, change of routine: these are all reasons. (Knowing why does not make us feel better!)

I recently attended a meditation retreat where people were surreptitiously speaking in hushed tones and looking guilty. One was saying she always becomes constipated on these retreats, and the others were nodding. Several said that they had resigned themselves to suffering for the length of the retreat. I remembered that I also had this experience the last few times I had come there.

This had my attention. I studied the food, which was served buffet style. This is a great place, and the food is excellent. Was there too much starch, fat, salt, or sugar? No, the food is well planned and prepared. I found a wonderful combination of fresh salads, homemade breads, vegetables, and fish, poultry, or meat at every meal. There was plenty of fiber. The problem wasn't the food (although some people will lock up whenever their diet changes, regardless of food quality).

Knowing that travel can dry us, I increased my

consumption of water. Every waking hour, I drank at least 8–10 ounces of water. (That resulted in more than a gallon of water a day! You have to know I was determined.) Well, soon I was very well hydrated and visiting the bathroom every hour. I also was able to move my bowels. Drinking more water really helped! Others tried it and experienced similar results. Still, I had to strain.

Every day, we had a movement class. One day, we were making drumming noises, rhythmically patting our lower abdomens. After doing this for 5 or 10 minutes, I began feeling movement in my bowels. That day, there was no strain. Of course! Here we were, like at most conferences, spending our time sitting. In a way, stagnating. Add movement, and the stagnation clears. Interestingly, long walks were not enough (although they often do the trick). Our bodies required more direct stimulation.

Herbal Recommendations

If you are planning a trip and you commonly become constipated, pack a remedy for it. My favorite herbal remedy for travel is *cascara sagrada*, a bowel tonic. It works best in tincture form. The standard dose is 1–3 droppersful, taken before bed. If you have taken that dose and do not move your bowels the following day, I recommend increasing the number of doses to 2 times per day and, if necessary, to 3 times per day. Substitutes for cascara sagrada include *rhubarb* and *senna*; both are available in tincture form. Take them at the same dose and frequency as cascara sagrada.

Ground psyllium seed is the herb of choice for many people. It is a pure bulking agent that is the primary ingredient of Metamucil, the popular over-the-counter preparation for constipation. For many people, psyllium helps compensate for the reduced fiber in travel food. People find that it softens their stool and makes it easier to expel. **Caution: You MUST drink sufficient water or psyllium can cause bloating!** This is NOT the herb for you if you refuse to drink water. To take, stir 1 rounded teaspoonful into 8 ounces of water or juice and drink immediately. (If you stir and wait, the water or juice will solidify.) Take 1–3 times per day. Many people add this to their protein drink or to their morning juice.

Triphala is a famous remedy from the Ayurvedic tradition (the Asian Indian medical system) that normalizes bowel function through its balancing effect on the three doshas (the three Ayurvedic metaphors that describe body function). Not surprisingly, it is the most widely used herbal formula in the world and is used by millions of people every day. It also is a bowel tonic that strengthens bowel function and may be taken safely for years. Take 2 capsules 1–3 times per day. Alternatively, stir 1 teaspoon of triphala powder into 8 ounces of hot water, wait until the powder settles to the bottom, and drink the water. Feel free to add more water and reuse the powder a second time that day. The dose of the powder is 1 teaspoon taken 2 times per day.

Homeopathic Remedies

If you possess a "shy" colon — you might move your bowels if only everyone would leave you alone for an hour — try homeopathic *Natrum mur. 30c*. The number of doses varies: dissolve 1–3 pellets beneath your tongue 1–3 times per day. You also can use this remedy for cold sores.

If your constipation results from over-indulging in food or drink, try homeopathic *Nux vomica 30c*. Dissolve 1–3 pellets beneath your tongue 1–3 times per day. You also can use this remedy for hangovers.

If your constipation is from dehydration, try homeopathic *Bryonia 30c*. Dissolve 1–3 pellets beneath your tongue 1–3 times per day. Try it for dry, hacking coughs. See "Choosing Homeopathic Remedies," page 12.

Food Recommendations

The best food remedy for constipation is *prune juice or stewed prunes*. For many people, 6 ounces (juice glass) or 8 ounces (water glass) of prune juice, once a day, is sufficient. Many hotels and restau-

CONSTIPATION

rants offer stewed prunes at breakfast: try to eat at least 8–10 prunes. Alternatively, try *figs*. In season, you can find them fresh — they are scrumptious! Many grocery stores stock both dried prunes and dried figs; eat 8–12 a day of either. Most groceries carry prune juice in quart bottles or in 6 packs of 6 ounce cans. The quart bottles provide a better value if you have access to refrigeration.

Generally, to relieve constipation, *increase fiber and decrease refined starches*. For some people, the choice of a bran muffin in place of a bagel, biscuit, or piece of toast will be sufficient. Some people like to carry bran to stir into their cereal or flax seeds to top their salad. Eating fresh fruits and vegetables adds fiber to the diet. Some people find that eating a whole grapefruit in the morning guarantees a bowel movement the next morning. Grapefruit juice usually does not have the same effect. **Caution: Cooked fruits and vegetables are safer travel choices than raw, especially in areas where water quality or restaurant cleanliness is poor.** See the "Parasites" chapter for more information.

Avoiding certain foods greatly aids in elimination. Highly refined foods, such as bread, cake, and cookies literally can gum up the works. White flour mixed with water and a pinch of salt dries into an incredible, immovable glue. As I read lists of ingredients, I've often wondered about how we metabolize this very same combination. From personal experience and that of many travelers, eating fewer breads, cakes, and cookies helps to keep things moving. Avoiding white rice, pasta, instant mashed potatoes, instant oatmeal, and instant "any starch" also will help.

Coffee stimulates bowel function. If you always drink coffee while at home but NOT when you travel, and you become constipated when you travel, the lack of coffee may be the source of your constipation. You may need to compensate — try one of the herbal remedies listed at the top of this section.

Proper food combining aids digestion and thereby relieves constipation. Whole books have been written on the details of this subject, and you may wish to read one. For our purposes, the "rules" of food combining are simple:

- Do not eat starch (potatoes, rice, and other grain products) with animal protein. This means no meat sandwiches. No meat and potatoes. No chicken and rice.
- Eat starch with non-starchy vegetables.
- Eat protein with non-starchy vegetables, such as a grilled chicken salad.
- Eat fat with protein.
- Do not eat fat with starch.
- Eat fruits as a snack or as a separate meal.

Following the food combining rules is easier

CONSTIPATION

than it looks. Proper food combining may eliminate constipation, and it usually eliminates gas — another travel issue.

Private Time

Give yourself *private time* for elimination. Many people have a "shy" colon; they will not eliminate on demand and certainly not in the presence of others. Others simply need sufficient time, which often seems unavailable while traveling. If this is you, find the time and the place where you have what you need. For some, this means going down to the hotel lobby early in the morning for a private walk. No one needs to know how you spend most of your walk time.

Self Massage

Circular tummy rubs, following the direction of the colon, may assist with elimination. Your colon begins near the crease between your right hip and thigh, travels up towards your ribs, goes horizontally from the right to the left and travels down along your left side, towards the center and then out. Using the palm of one or both hands, make clockwise circles on your abdomen, following the course of colon. Doing this for 5 or more minutes per day adds energy to your system, may counter the stagnation of prolonged sitting, is pleasant, and costs nothing.

Herbal Remedies in the Wilderness

Prepare your own psyllium seed substitute from the seeds of the *plantain* plant! (*Plantago psyllium*, a kind of plantain, is the only source of psyllium seeds, but the seeds of other plantain species will work almost as well.) Soak 1 or more teaspoons of the seeds in a cup of water overnight and drink or add to cooking liquids the next day. Alternatively, chew and swallow 1 teaspoon of the seeds or simmer as a tea. Take 1–3 times per day.

The roots of *dandelion*, *yellow dock*, or *Solomon's seal* plants, found widely throughout the United States, serve as laxatives. Simmer 1 tablespoon of the cleaned and minced root in 2 cups of water for 20–30 minutes, cool, and drink 2–3 times per day.

CONSTIPATION

Constipation Summary of Remedies

To avoid or eliminate constipation:

- Water: Drink 64–128 ounces per day.
- Exercise: Walking, running, yoga, tai chi, ANYTHING that keeps you moving.
- Herbs: Take cascara sagrada, psyllium seed, triphala. Other herbs include senna and rhubarb.
- Foods: Eat prunes, figs, or grapefruit.
  Avoid starch, salt, and sugar.
  Increase fiber.
  Combine foods properly.
- Find privacy and time for elimination.
- Perform circular tummy rubs.

Top choices of packable constipation remedies (you only need one):

- Cascara sagrada tincture.
- Triphala capsules.
- Homeopathic: Natrum mur. 30c, Nux vomica 30c, Bryonia 30c.

Top wilderness choices:

- Plantain seed.
- Dandelion root.
- Yellow dock root.
- Solomon's seal root.

CONSTIPATION

DIARRHEA

Imagine you and the family have finally gone on that much needed vacation. You have driven to a beautiful park. You hiked for six hours, carrying all your gear to your campsite, where you plan to relax for the next week. You set up your tent, you hang your hammock…and your 4-year-old daughter, whom you carried most of the way, informs you she has diarrhea. Bad diarrhea.

What are you going to do?

Diarrhea can spoil any trip. People experiencing it — most of us have — can be totally miserable! In a youngster, it can be especially debilitating. Diarrhea is very dehydrating and requires continual drinking of large quantities of water to avoid the extreme fatigue that often accompanies it. It can prevent the sufferer and her companions from any travel beyond the nearest bathroom or rest station. Left to run its course, diarrhea easily can continue for 48–72 hours.

Avoiding Diarrhea

See "Reducing the Likelihood of Parasite Infestation" in the "Parasites" chapter.

Dealing with Diarrhea

Luckily, anywhere in the world, you can find

great remedies for diarrhea that work. You can purchase herbal or pharmaceutical remedies for your travel kit, you can find food remedies in restaurants and food stores, and you can even find remedies in the woods.

Regardless of how you choose to treat your diarrhea, drink water. *Drink a lot of water.* Drink more than you feel comfortable drinking. Why? Diarrhea is one of the most dehydrating conditions you can experience. The dehydration is responsible for much of the fatigue and will lengthen your recovery. Diarrhea can be life-threatening, especially for a child or an elderly person. So drink!

Food and Diarrhea

What can you safely eat if you suddenly have diarrhea? Certain foods work extremely well. Remember the *BRAT diet* for children? Consisting of bananas, (white) rice, apples (grated and allowed to brown), and toast (burnt), this diet includes two excellent remedies. *Burnt toast*, available around the world, is a form of charcoal, and will both detoxify your system and eventually stop diarrhea. (See section below on "Charcoal.") Eat 1 or 2 slices. The toast is too dry? Feel free to dunk it in *black tea*. Tea contains tannic acid, which also will help stop diarrhea. *White rice* will solidify your stool. So will *whey protein*, which is often used by bodybuilders as a supplement and is now widely available. While you are suffering from diarrhea, avoid all foods that clear constipation. Avoid raw fruits, vegetables, and juices and avoid prunes and figs. Eat more starchy food, such as cooked potatoes, rice, and other grains, and eat less fat. Eliminate coffee — it stimulates bowel activity.

Umeboshi plum is a wonderful Oriental remedy for diarrhea. Studies show that constituents of umeboshi are anti-bacterial. Umeboshi works particularly well at eliminating dysentery and the staphylococci bacteria. Purchase prepared umeboshi (paste or whole plums) in Oriental stores or in natural food stores in the macrobiotic section. Although umeboshi usually is used as a very salty and sour condiment, you will use it as a medicinal food. Take approximately 1 teaspoon — or 1 plum — every two hours until the diarrhea clears. You also can take umeboshi mashed into rice or simmered in tea.

Mung beans and mung bean tea are another remedy for diarrhea. Mung beans are detoxifying and may be used to treat food poisoning, dysentery, pesticide poisoning, boils, hot skin rashes, and heat exhaustion. They are especially useful at clearing diarrhea accompanied by fever or sweating. Small and olive-green, mung beans are the unsprouted version of bean sprouts. Purchase them dried in Oriental food stores or in natural food stores. To cook, simmer 1 cup of mung beans in 4 cups of water for $1^1/2$ hours (you may begin sipping the simmered water after only 20 minutes). Both the cooked beans and the water clear diarrhea. Although this may sound like too mild a remedy, I know of cases where mung bean tea did the trick when nothing else worked. Drink half a cup to 1 cup per hour. When you feel strong enough for solid food, eat the beans.

Drugstore Remedy

Most pharmacists recommend a product called *Imodium*. Follow directions on the label. Often, 1 pill is sufficient to stop diarrhea. It is reliable, and many seasoned travelers recommend it.

Herbal Remedies

I recommend that travelers with a tendency towards diarrhea obtain the herb *blackberry root* in a 1 ounce tincture bottle. It is gentle and VERY effective. Stop taking it once the diarrhea stops — you risk constipation if you continue taking it too long. It is available at health food stores. Alternatively, try *cranesbill*, also known as geranium or wild geranium, in a 1 ounce tincture bottle. Take 1 dropperful of either blackberry root or cranesbill every half hour until diarrhea stops.

If diarrhea follows exposure to cold (you go

swimming on a cold day and you don't cover up after coming out of the water), try *ginger* from your kit. (See the "Making a Travel Kit" section.) Chances are the ginger will sufficiently heat your chilled system and the diarrhea will end. Quickly.

Homeopathic Remedies

In some areas, homeopathic remedies are the easiest medicines to find, and the little plastic vials that hold tiny pellets are convenient to carry. I recommend the potency of 30c. See "Choosing Homeopathic Remedies," page 12. *Nux vomica* works for the overworked, irritable, and chilly traveler who has been eating too much and too many heavy foods and for the person who feels the frequent urge to defecate but often cannot. It is good for the workaholic with alternating diarrhea and constipation. Did you overeat? Did you drink too much? Try Nux vomica. Take 1–3 of the tiny pellets every 15 minutes until symptoms cease, and take again if symptoms return.

Arsenicum works for the exhausted and restless traveler with explosive diarrhea and vomiting. It's also a good choice for food poisoning or when you feel pain at your stomach. Try Arsenicum whenever you have both diarrhea and vomiting. *Gelsemium* helps the nervous traveler who knows her diarrhea results from anxiety — it's the performer's remedy.

Pulsatilla helps those who have over-indulged in rich foods who have diarrhea at night. *Sulphur* helps travelers with "cock's crow" diarrhea, the kind that occurs painlessly at dawn. For all of the homeopathic remedies for diarrhea, take 1–3 of the tiny pills every 15 minutes until the symptoms cease and again if symptoms return.

Charcoal

Charcoal is a VERY GOOD remedy for all sorts of food and chemical poisoning. It is used by a wide range of healthcare providers, including medical doctors, herbalists, and naturopathic physicians. Unlike Imodium or cranesbill, charcoal not only stops the diarrhea but also helps to eliminate the toxicity that may be the cause. Think of charcoal as acting much like a sponge that attracts and holds on to many times its own weight in toxins. The toxins bind to the charcoal and are then eliminated through the colon.

Activated charcoal is the most compact form. You can find activated charcoal in pills and capsules and in powdered form in pharmacies and health food stores. Charcoal capsules work well for many people and are easily packed. The dose is 2 capsules every 1–2 hours until diarrhea stops, then 2 capsules 1–3 times per day. In extreme cases, you can take more. To use the powdered form, stir 1–3 teaspoons of charcoal in 1 cup of water and swallow.

Need it NOW? Make your own vegetable charcoal by burning bread, popcorn, or any starchy food to a crisp. To be most effective, the food should be deep black and snap when you break it. Vegetable charcoal works very well, but you will need to use more of it than you would the activated charcoal. Use 1–2 tablespoons of the vegetable charcoal for each dose. To make it easier to take, crush it and dissolve in water.

Charcoal will temporarily turn your teeth, gums, and tongue black! Just continue rinsing with water. It also will turn your stool black — so don't panic. And when charcoal first goes through your system, it provides additional force to your bowel movement.

Clay

Bentonite clay, available in health food stores, will slow and later stop diarrhea while helping to detoxify the colon. The dose is 1 tablespoon dissolved in water. This remedy is often taken long term to help clear toxicity in the body, but it also works well short term. If you choose to gather your own clay, you must heat it for at least 1 hour in a 225–250 degree oven to kill the likely bacteria in the clay. No, I don't know how to find edible clay in the wild. You are on your own if you choose to gather

DIARRHEA

clay. Better yet, if you are in an area known for this use of clay, seek out an expert. Like charcoal, clay is cheap, readily available, and works very well.

Diarrhea in the Wilderness

What if you are in the wild? The root (preferably) or leaf from any *blackberry or raspberry vine* is VERY effective. I recommend making a tea by cleaning and simmering a quarter cup to half cup of the cut-up root or leaf in 2 cups of water for at least 10–30 minutes. While you are waiting, chewing a piece of the cleaned root will help. *Wild strawberry* root and leaf and *blueberry* leaf also work but are slightly less effective. Prepare them the same way that you prepare the blackberry and raspberry tea. Drink a cup of tea per hour until the diarrhea clears.

Can't find any bramble/berry plants? *Kudzu*, which grows abundantly throughout the southeastern United States, is also effective. Simmer 2 tablespoons of the cleaned, cut-up root in 2 cups of water. Plan on drinking half a cup of the liquid per hour until the diarrhea stops. By the way, the kudzu root or flower are both great remedies for hangovers — make the tea described above.

You are in the woods? *Burn the wood* from trees, shrubs, or other plant matter. Use a known plant, preferably one that is used medicinally or for food. Rely on your field guide. Some plants may be toxic — don't use one you can't identify. Many hardwoods, including oaks, maples, and conifers are good choices. Burning any edible starch and eating the *charcoal* will work. Starch includes rice, potatoes, grits, bread, and corn products. You also can char and eat kudzu root if you are in the southeastern United States. **Caution: Do not use the kind of charcoal used for grilling or starting fires.**

Do you see any *weeping willow* trees? Easily identified, the bark of the willow tree is high in tannic acid, a known astringent. Willow bark tea is a good remedy for diarrhea. The inner bark of the *white oak* (white oak is especially good, other oaks will work) also makes a tea that will stop diarrhea. Prune some small branches and cut the inner bark in strips. Simmer approximately 1 tablespoon of bark in $1^1/2$ cups of water for 20–30 minutes. Drink $1/2$ cup every 30 minutes.

Diarrhea Summary of Remedies

To avoid or eliminate diarrhea:

- Water: Drink plenty of pure water.
- Foods: White rice.
                      B.R.A.T. diet. (bananas, white rice,
                      (brown) grated apple, burned toast).
                      Tea and toast.
                      High starch, low fat diet.
                      Whey protein.
                      Umeboshi plum.
                      Mung beans and mung bean juice.
- Herbs: Blackberry root or cranesbill (also
                      known as geranium).
                      Ginger (if diarrhea resulted from
                      exposure to cold).
- Homeopathics: Nux vomica 30c.
                      Arsenicum 30c.
                      Gelsemium 30c.
                      Pulsatilla 30c.
                      Sulphur 30c.
- Other: Activated charcoal.
                      Bentonite clay.
- Drugs: Imodium.

Top choices of packable remedies:

- Blackberry root tincture.
- Activated charcoal capsules.
- Nux vomica 30c.
- Imodium.

Top wilderness remedies:

- Wild blackberry, raspberry, or strawberry leaf and
  root.
- White oak tree inner bark.
- Willow tree bark.
- Charcoal (not the kind used for grilling or for starting
  fires!)

FAST FOOD

You are traveling cross country. You are trying your best to stay alert, stay awake, and arrive at your destination on time. You have food in the car with you to eat when you are bored. Your top choices for car food include your favorite chips, nuts, and sweet snacks. When you MUST pull over for a bathroom break, you choose coffee or soda to replenish your fluids and limit your choice of restaurants to those within 0.2 miles of the exit.

You notice how tired you become just from driving. Hmmm. Could your choices of food and drink make you tired? Sugar, salt, grease, and chocolate — the four major (car) food groups — taken continually for hours on end will put anyone to sleep. When you get really sleepy, you pull over for a cup of coffee — caffeine!

Even if you don't eat in the car, most travelers choose fast food restaurants to save time and money when traveling. You choose your food while standing in a line that moves too slowly and place your order with a bored, indifferent, or impatient server. You eat your food, likely high in fat, salt, and sugar, as quickly as possible, dump the remains in the trash, and rush back to your car.

Consider traveling a little farther to find restaurants that serve more than just fast food. Look for places that cook food to order. Local, non-chain restaurants sometimes provide "home cooking" that includes locally grown produce.

Finding Food on the Road

My mother once asked me, "So, what SHOULD I eat? Am I stuck with carrying baggies full of banana chips?" Actually, unsweetened banana chips provide a good alternative to many snack foods, and I advised Mom to carry them. Luckily, she can find many other foods to eat during her travels.

The key to selecting travel food lies in making the best choices among alternatives. We all need a balance of protein, fat, and carbohydrates. Generally, if you eat at least 5 ounces of meat, fish, or poultry per day, you will be eating the minimum requirement of fats and protein. If you eat at least 8 ounces of beans or bean products such as tofu, you will be meeting the minimum requirement for protein but may need to supplement your fats. If you eat at least 5 half-cup portions of fruits or vegetables each day, you will be meeting the minimum requirement for carbohydrates. For additional calories and energy, some people require grains such as rice, barley, or corn. (Grains are mostly carbohydrates, but contain protein and small — almost negligible —

FAST FOOD

amounts of fat.)

If you are eating in a fast food restaurant, consciously choose to make healthy choices. When possible, reduce fat, chemicals, sugar, and salt and increase the fiber. Eat food in as close to its whole form as possible. Say NO to fried food.

CARBOHYDRATES are not all equal. As a general rule, the less processed, the greater the nutritional value. Bread, particularly highly processed white bread or white sandwich rolls, are not a substitute for whole grains, fruits, or vegetables. *Given the choice, always choose the less processed food.* Choose whole or steel-cut oats over instant oats. Choose brown rice over white rice. Choose regular grits over instant grits. Given a choice between baked potato and french fries, choose the baked potato. If you must have starch and you can choose only fried potatoes or a bag of potato chips, choose the fried potatoes. But know that you are choosing a food that is more fat than carbohydrate.

What about the bun or bread? Toss it! We are not talking about high quality breads that sustain life. They are highly salted and sugared flour-foods that have been stripped of fiber. Often, the bread is smeared with additional fat in the form of margarine, butter, or mayonnaise. Many people find that they feel more awake if they skip the roll or the bread. Some find that they are less prone to stomach upsets. Try it. If you must have bread, choose a whole grain bread.

Do *look for more vegetables*. Sure, in some places, you will be limited to lettuce and tomato — ask for an additional portion and expect to pay for it. Order side dishes of vegetables — you will feel better. Salad is a great choice, but avoid lunch meats (ham, salami, etc.) and high fat salad dressings.

FATS are not all equal. While some fats promote health and well-being, others literally make us sick! Reports from leading medical institutions and health groups indicate that trans fats are unhealthy and contribute to heart disease. Many trans fats or trans fatty acids are liquid fats that have been artificially solidified to improve taste or mouth-feel. (A very small portion of animal fats may contain trans fats.) Most fats that are liquid at room temperature do not contain trans fats.

The most common trans fats are most margarines and all solid vegetable shortenings. Most fried food is high in trans fat. (Remember those fried potatoes?) So are most commercial pastries, such as cinnamon rolls and fried pies. Read the labels. All "hydrogenated" or "partially hydrogenated fats" include trans fatty acids. Don't eat them.

Eat healthy fats instead. We need fat to survive. Recommended fat foods include avocado, seeds, nuts, and coconut. For meat eaters, lean cuts of

meat, fish, and poultry contain fat. Many nutrition-
ists recommend the daily consumption of 2 tablespoons of freshly ground flax seed or flax seed oil,
which contains healthful omega-3 fatty acids
Because flax seed oil is highly perishable and must
be kept refrigerated, it is not a good travel food. (Try
the flax seed oil capsules when you travel — they are
easy to carry, but you'll need to take 12 capsules
to equal 1 tablespoon of the oil! Whole flax seeds
travel well, but you will need to grind them to
obtain the full omega-3 fatty acid benefits.) For
cooking and salad dressings, olive oil is the time-
tested healthy choice. I choose butter, preferably
organic butter, over margarine.

PROTEINS are not all equal. If you want chick-
en and have a choice between grilled chicken or
breaded and fried chicken, choose the grilled. (The
cook likely uses trans fats in the deep fat fryer.) If
you have a choice between fried chopped and
formed chicken or fried whole pieces of chicken,
choose the whole pieces. If you want to have fish
and the only choice is breaded and fried, feel free to
scrape off the breading and eat the fish. When possible, *choose organic or free range meats and cold
water fishes*. I choose wild caught fish over farm
raised fish due to superior taste and nutritional
value.

Bring Your Own Snacks

Bring some bars. I like bringing high quality protein bars or meal replacement bars with me when I travel. Protein bars have the advantage of easy packability and they stay fresh for long periods. I am quite particular about which protein bars I eat. (Two I enjoy are Boulder Bars and Balance Bars.) I suggest that you be particular too! I don't buy bars that contain artificial sweeteners such as aspartame (also known as NutraSweet) or Sweet 'n Low. I consider those substances dangerous, and I refuse to eat them. I also look for bars with at least 15 grams of protein per serving and whole fruit sweeteners.

Consider carrying fruit. Fresh fruit is the least processed but spoils more easily. Caution: In areas where tap water quality is uncertain, stick to fruit you peel yourself (do not eat the peel!) or wash and soak the fruit first in pure (bottled or boiled) water to which you have added 10–20 drops of grapefruit seed extract. A potent but digestible antiseptic, grapefruit seed extract is available at health food stores.

Unsweetened juices provide a healthy snack — consider 1 cup of juice as the rough equivalent of 1 piece of fruit. Limit juice intake to 1 cup per day. **Caution: Although fresh, non-pasteurized juices provide outstanding nutrition, insist on pasteurized for people with compromised immune systems.**

Easily available dried fruits include raisins, prunes, apples, pears, cranberries, and banana chips among others! About $1/2$ cup equals 1 portion.

How about vegetables? VEGETABLES? Sure! An increasing variety of freeze-dried vegetables have become available in natural food and specialty food shops. Freeze-dried carrots, corn, and peas are all tasty. Also, consider bringing freeze-dried soups and dips that easily reconstitute with water: try black beans, refried beans, hummus (chick peas), lentils, and split peas. They're easy to carry.

Nuts and seeds provide an excellent source of protein and fat. I recommend low or no salt types. (Salted ones provide too much salt.) Roasted nuts and seeds are more easily digested than raw ones. Consider sunflower seeds, pumpkin seeds, soy nuts, and all nuts except peanuts. Why no peanuts? A VERY high percentage of people are allergic to them. Also, aflatoxin, a toxic mold, is common on peanuts. NOTE: Some organic peanuts are tested for aflatoxin — check the label. One-eighth to one-quarter cup of nuts or seeds equals 1 portion.

Grains, such as unsweetened puffed grains, can provide a tasty snack, especially with a nut or fruit butter. Brown rice or popcorn cakes are widely available, pack well, and are easily stored, but eat them with caution if you are carbohydrate sensitive. Do read the label before purchasing — some contain

FAST FOOD

lots of sodium or sugar.

Consider homemade granola and granola bars. Made from whole oats, nuts and seeds, a whole sweetener and dried fruits, granola makes an excellent and easily packed snack.

Bring bottled water! You'll stay hydrated and you won't be as tempted by sodas and other sweetened drinks.

Fast Food Summary

Finding food on the road:

- Select the best choices among alternatives:
  Less processed rather than more processed.
  Grilled rather than fried.
  Fresh rather than packaged, processed, or stored.

- Balance proteins, fats, and carbohydrates.

- Choose healthy fats:
  Avocado, olive oil, flax seed, and flax seed oil;
    butter rather than margarine.
  Avoid fried foods and commercial pastries.

- Avoid chemicals, artificial sweeteners, sugar, and salt.

Bring your own snacks:

- Protein and meal replacement bars.

- Fruit: fresh, dried, and juice.

- Vegetables: fresh and dried.

- Nuts and seeds.

- Bottled water.

FOOT PROBLEMS

Years ago as a courtroom attorney, I wore the "uniform": navy blue suit, pumps with 2 inch heels, stockings. Although I lived in Atlanta, I was representing my Washington, D.C. client in a case in Orange County, California. The day before our trial, I awakened at 6 a.m., went for a run, changed into my "uniform," and was at work by 8. Still wearing stockings and heels, I met my client at the airport. (What was I thinking?) Like everyone else, we walked the mile in the airport to our plane. We flew to Dallas, where we had a two-hour layover and changed planes. We walked the mile to the next plane, me still in stockings and heels, and flew to LAX. Upon arrival we walked through the airport to baggage claim, dragged our luggage to ground transportation, and stood in line for the rental car. (My swollen feet!) We drove over an hour to our Orange County destination. By now, my swollen feet were on fire and my shoes were cutting into my feet. I was afraid to take off my shoes in the car — what if I couldn't get them back on? We arrived at the federal courthouse and admired the beautiful and incredibly hard marble floors. Every step hurt.

We walked (why wasn't I wearing sneakers?) to the file clerk's office and stood in line. Then we walked to the judge's office and waited, standing, for a clerk. I could barely concentrate.

I was wearing very sensible shoes that were well broken-in. Selbys. Navy blue, medium heel, wide toe. It didn't matter. By the end of the day all I could think of was the pain. When I finally got to my hotel room I gently tried to remove my shoes. They didn't budge. I looked. My feet were bulging out and gripping the shoes. I wrenched one shoe off and quickly began massaging my swollen and aching foot. (Why do we wear these things?!?) There were deep creases where the shoe cut me. The creases burned. My arches ached.

Today, older and wiser, you couldn't pay me to wear heels through three airports and on two planes. Wearing heels or any tight or ill-fitting shoes will guarantee aching feet on an extended trip. Given the right conditions, even comfortably clad feet will swell and hurt.

General Advice

Avoid getting sore feet. Assume that you will walk more than usual when traveling so wear comfortable shoes with adequate support. Shoes that pinch, bind, rub, or squeeze do not qualify — leave them home. If you need such shoes for your job or a special event, carry them and change your shoes after you arrive.

Wear the recommended foot gear for your travel. I still remember the woman at the bottom of the Grand Canyon with the most amazing blisters. She had hiked down the day before wearing sandals. SANDALS! The recommended footgear was heavy duty hiking boots with two pairs of socks. Needless to say, she couldn't hike anywhere. (Wearing sandals, she also risked twisting an ankle, sunburn, and snake, scorpion, and other bites.) She was lucky, all she had was blisters. She eventually was airlifted out of the canyon at tremendous expense (to her).

If you wear special shoe *inserts or insoles*, be sure to bring them and wear them. Magnetic insoles, available in drugstores, natural food stores, and through the Nikken company, reduce foot fatigue and aches for many people. I think they are great! Cushioned insoles, which are very inexpensive and available at drugstores and supermarkets, can help.

Keep your feet dry. Travel often entails keeping our shoes on for longer periods of time so our feet don't air out. When camping, many people keep their socks on even after removing their shoes. The socks retain moisture and the feet stay damp. If you feel the need to constantly wear socks, when you remove your shoes, dry your feet, powder them, and change your socks.

FOOT PROBLEMS

Be aware that your feet sweat. To keep your feet drier, *air your feet* at regular intervals. To absorb added moisture, powder your feet with *marshmallow root powder*, *talcum powder*, or *cornstarch*. Available in health food stores, marshmallow root smoothes away friction while absorbing moisture. Keeping your feet dry will reduce the likelihood of hot spots, blisters, and athlete's foot.

Use moleskin. Stick self-adhesive moleskin on spots that normally become sore to prevent blistering. When walking, hiking, or trekking, STOP and apply moleskin as soon as you feel a sore or hot spot developing — you will avoid most blisters this way.

Try orthotics. If you chronically suffer from sore and aching feet, you may benefit from orthotics. Orthotics are shoe inserts that are customized for your feet. They can eliminate many foot and posture problems — greatly improving the quality of your travel. Podiatrists and many chiropractors prescribe orthotics; you may wish to speak with a podiatrist or chiropractor to find if orthotics are right for you.

Elevate your feet. Placing your feet above the level of your heart puts gravity to work for you. You can reduce swelling at no expense and your feet will feel so much better. Raising your feet even a little will help soothe tired feet. When you anticipate a long day or when your feet already hurt, use a footrest. On plane trips, arrange your under-seat luggage or pillows to create a footrest and place your feet on top of it. It will help!

Massage your feet with a ball. Sure, I'd love to have a massage therapist nurture my feet, but that is not always convenient. Take any small ball — a golf ball or a tennis ball — place it under your foot and apply pressure to it while rolling it back and forth and around. Don't press so hard that you bruise yourself. Within moments your foot will begin to tingle. Continue your massage for a few seconds more and switch feet. Ahhh.

Get a professional pedicure before you travel. A friend does this prior to all trips, and she swears by it! The pedicurist trims and shapes all the nails, softens calluses, and finishes with a foot massage. Nail color is included. (I'm thinking about this for my next trip….)

Herbs

Several years ago I attended my nephew's Bar Mitzvah at a beautiful country inn in New Hampshire. It was the end of a long day and my father, the original party animal, was moving slowly and wincing. I pulled him aside and he reluctantly told me that he had left his prescription diuretic, Lasix, at home. He pulled up his pants legs — his ankles were swollen like melons! He was afraid to take off his shoes because he was certain he'd never get them back on. We were miles away from the nearest store. He agreed to try an herb — anything to reduce the swelling.

I follow a simple rule in cases like this, "The herb you need is in your own backyard" (or in the kitchen or on the hotel grounds). I went outside for a walk. Dandelion plants were everywhere, and within moments I had a handful of *dandelion leaf.* I rinsed the leaf in the bathroom sink, tore it into small pieces, and crushed it with a spoon inside Dad's room mug. I added boiling water from the kitchen, steeped it for 5 minutes, stirred, and gave Dad his tea. Fifteen minutes later, he grinned and walked to the bathroom. He drank about 4 mugs per day, was able to delay using Lasix until he returned home, and eliminated his ankle swelling.

Interestingly, when we returned to my parents' home in New Jersey, I noticed the weed *plantain* was growing everywhere. Plantain is another excellent diuretic that can be prepared the same way as dandelion leaf. An herb Dad needed really does grow in his yard.

If you are retaining water, you may wish to take 1 dropperful of dandelion leaf tincture (not the root) or 1 teaspoon of the tea steeped or simmered in 1 cup of water for 5 minutes, 3 times per day. You may wish to gather your own fresh leaf and drink the tea like my father did. It will send you to the bathroom, so be sure to continue drinking your water. Dandelion leaf is a remarkable diuretic because it is so gentle and so effective. It even contains its own potassium.

Sometimes your feet ache and you want to put something on them. *Witch hazel* is an excellent, astringent remedy that relieves sore and achy feet. Buy witch hazel liquid from the drugstore or natural food store and apply it directly to those aching feet. Use enough to moisten the skin, rub it in, and let your feet and ankles air dry. Long term daily use will shrink varicose veins — it really works!

You say you don't have any witch hazel? Soak your feet in *ginger tea*. Ginger's mildly stimulating effect gets your foot fluids moving, thereby relieving swelling and pain. Another good foot bath choice is *Epsom salts*. Dissolve a cup of Epsom salts in 1–2 quarts of hot water and soak your feet in the solution. Add 1–2 drops of peppermint or lavender essential oil to the foot bath for a spa-like experience.

Homeopathics

Homeopathic *Arnica* taken internally (dissolve 1–4 of the tiny sugar pills beneath your tongue) or *Arnica gel or cream* smoothed on your feet reduces soreness. Use at the beginning of your travel day to reduce swelling and pain. Continue taking Arnica internally every 20 minutes while you are feeling pain and 3 times a day while traveling without pain. Feel free to use both the internal and external forms. **Caution: Don't use Arnica externally on broken skin.**

If you get swollen feet and Arnica just isn't enough, you might want to try homeopathic witch hazel, *Hamamelis*. (Any potency of or less than 10x or 10c will be fine.) Take 4 of the tiny pills at the beginning of the day and repeat this dose for a total of at least 3 times per day. You may take this remedy every 20 minutes to reduce the pain of aching feet. See "Choosing Homeopathic Remedies," page 12.

Essential Oils

Essential oils are the BEST when it comes to feet! One drop of *peppermint essential oil* in cool water makes a refreshing foot bath for hot and aching feet. Try a *lavender essential oil* compress by adding 5 drops to a moistened handkerchief and massage upwards from your feet to your calves. This is a great remedy for airline foot swelling, and you can do it on the plane.

Food Choices for Sore or Swollen Feet

If your swollen feet are the simple result of water retention, *stop eating salt*. This can be difficult when traveling because so many prepared foods are made with large amounts of salt. Still, you can reduce your salt consumption by putting down the salt shaker. Also, avoid eating high-salt foods such as salted nuts, salty chips, canned soups, canned tomato juice, and many sauces. Increase your consumption of water to flush your system and reduce water retention.

Dandelion leaf, which is available in many areas as a salad or cooked green, is a potent diuretic that will reduce swelling. *Nettles*, which may be cooked as a pot herb (cook it in soup as a green) or simmered for 20 minutes for tea, is another natural diuretic. Pick your own (but wear gloves, nettles sting until dried or cooked!). Or find nettle leaf tea at a natural food store. *Watermelon*, or a tea made from a handful of the seeds simmered in 2 cups of water for 20 minutes, will clear excess water and will cool you down. *Cooked barley or barley tea*, made by simmering a quarter cup of barley in 2 cups of water for 20 minutes, will reduce swollen feet and ankles. Drink 2–4 cups per day.

Athlete's Foot, Fungus, and Yeast

Athlete's foot, fungus, and yeast, when on the feet, are three ways of saying the same thing. These are common problems for many people that are exacerbated by travel. Yeast thrives on dampness so if your feet stay damp you are inviting yeast. Keep your feet dry with *marshmallow root powder*, *cornstarch*, or *talcum powder*, and read the suggestions under "General Advice." If you have or tend to get athlete's foot, consider adding *baking soda* or *garlic powder* to your foot powder! Both eliminate yeast.

Cracking heels and torn skin between your toes are a sign of yeast. For relief, apply several drops of *tea tree oil* directly to your feet, full strength, 2–3 times per day. Or soak a cotton ball in tea tree oil and tape it to the area overnight. If your feet are sensitive to tea tree oil, dilute it by placing 15 drops of tea tree oil in 1–2 teaspoons (5–10 ml) of olive oil or another food grade oil. Alternatively, apply several drops of lavender essential oil, full strength, 2–3 times per day. You're in a remote area and can't obtain essential oils? Mash several *garlic cloves* (even available in the wilderness), and apply full strength for 1–2 hours or combine with cooking or massage oil overnight, apply, and cover with a sock. Overnight, the garlic cure can reduce even stubborn fungus problems, but full strength garlic WILL burn your feet if left in place for more than a few hours! It also will give you the worst case of garlic breath. (Eating a large handful of parsley reduces garlic breath.) Follow the garlic cure by applying lavender essential oil directly to the affected area. (Ten to 20 drops will cover the entire sole of your foot.)

Yellow or opaque finger nails or toe nails are a sign of yeast overgrowth. Apply a few drops of tea tree oil directly to the nail and the nail bed at least 2

FOOT PROBLEMS

times per day. This works remarkably well, especially when combined with an internal remedy (see below).

Know that foot fungus can be stubborn — it takes time to grow a new nail — and plan on continuing treatment for at least 6 months. To improve your results and reduce treatment time, treat yourself internally as well as externally. *Pau d'arco* is a tasty herb with outstanding anti-fungal qualities. Take 1 dropperful of the tincture 3 times per day or drink 1 cup of tea 3 times per day, made by simmering 3 tablespoons of herb in 4 cups of water for 30 minutes. Enjoy!

You can't find essential oils or herbs? Try vinegar for your foot fungus! *Vinegar* is available around the world and is inexpensive. Pour vinegar into a large bowl or small tub and soak your feet in it for at least 5 minutes daily. For quicker results, wrap your foot in a plastic bag filled with vinegar — a portable vinegar bath — and wear the bag for up to 24 hours. (Do the day-long bath only 1 time — repeated use can leach calcium from your body.) To speed the process, also take vinegar internally. Try to purchase apple cider vinegar — it is better for you and it is tasty. The dose is 1 teaspoon 3 times per day before meals, taken in $1/3$ cup of water. The combined internal and external approach speeds your healing.

When it comes to foot fungus, or fungus

anywhere in the body, natural remedies work as well or better than the highly priced and toxic prescription medications. You just need to take them consistently.

Stinky Feet

Essential oils can help clear the smell from stinky feet. Two drops of *cypress or lemongrass essential oil* added to your foot powder will naturally deodorize your feet. The cypress essential oil also helps relieve sore and achy feet.

If your feet smell, your socks and your shoes also smell. Be sure to change your socks at least once a day. Powder your feet with *baking soda* and sprinkle baking soda into your shoes each day. The baking soda absorbs odor.

FOOT PROBLEMS

Foot Problems Summary of Remedies

- Wear the recommended foot gear.
- Keep your feet dry.
- Air your feet at least once a day.
- Elevate your feet when possible.
- Massage. Roll your feet on a ball.
- Try magnetic or cushion insoles.
- Get a pedicure prior to travel.
- Diuretic herbs for excess water retention:
  Dandelion leaf.
  Nettle leaf.
  Plantain leaf.
- Footbaths:
  Epsom salts and essential oils.
  Ginger tea.
  Peppermint essential oil.
  Vinegar for athlete's foot.
- Witch hazel foot rubs.
- Homeopathic Arnica internally and externally.

FOOT PROBLEMS

INDIGESTION

You've waited all year for this trip. You've planned for months, read all the guidebooks, and now you have arrived at your destination. Your party is ready to explore, to find a great restaurant, or to just have fun. And YOU have a stomach ache. You feel ridiculous. You don't want to hold everyone back, you don't want to be the wet blanket in the group, but you really feel terrible. Everyone else is ready to rock and roll, and you would really rather sleep or watch TV and wait for your stomach to calm down.

Sound familiar? It is very common. At this point, slowing down and taking some time for yourself may be the best plan. It may not fit your schedule, but it certainly could help.

Breathe. This is a great time to just sit and BREATHE. Breathe slowly, focusing on your stomach, imagining that you are breathing in and out of your stomach. Close your eyes if you can. Think the word "calm" or "relax" or "easy" as you breathe. Five to ten minutes of quiet breathing may clear your indigestion and certainly will help you feel better. Can't do this in front of your group? I often imagine that hotel restrooms are filled with travelers doing their breathing and relaxation exercises. Don't feel shy. No one knows that you are breathing behind your locked stall door.

Stop eating. This may be a good time to take a break from eating. See how you feel. If missing a meal makes you queasy, try eating very lightly. Taking some tea with toast or crackers may settle your stomach. Try a little bit of soup or broth, but skip the cream or cheese. Eating lightly for 24 hours may be sufficient to eliminate your digestive woes.

Avoid fatty foods. Avoid all fried and high fat foods. Choose steamed or simmered vegetables instead of rich casseroles. Avoid buttery sauces. If you eat meat, eat small amounts that are lean. As a rule, red meat can be very difficult to digest. *Pay attention to how you combine your foods.* If you are eating more than a few ounces of protein, eat non-starchy vegetables such as a spinach, kale, or other greens and avoid bread, rice, and potatoes. You will feel better!

Travelers' Remedies

Several friends and clients, upon reading this section, told me that I missed the point. They said that when we travel, we CONSCIOUSLY indulge. They asked, rather pointedly, what can they take when they eat too much, drink too much, or generally indulge? For the hangover, heartburn, sour stomach, or acid indigestion caused by over-indulging, I recommend *Acidil* by Boiron. This is an outstanding homeopathic formula that combines Nux vomica 4c with homeopathic charcoal, black spruce, and yellow locust. Acidil works amazingly fast and amazingly well. Take 1 pill from the blister pack or 3 tiny pills from the tube pack every 15 minutes or until symptoms subside. Repeat as needed. Can't find Acidil? Substitute *Nux vomica 30c* and use the same dose and frequency. See "Choosing Homeopathic Remedies," page 12.

Essential Oils

I always carry a small (5 ml) bottle of *peppermint essential oil* with me. One drop (yes, only 1!) added to a glass of water helps to settle the stomach. Its mild sedating effect on the stomach eliminates nausea. This is a WONDERFUL remedy that works well for many people. It is my favorite conference remedy. It is easy to carry, smells nice, and works pretty well. Plus, there is plenty to share with all your friends.

Herbal Remedies

Many excellent indigestion remedies are found in the kitchen. Know that in an emergency, you usually can find what you need.

Yes, of course, *ginger.* Ginger candied,

powdered, fresh, tinctured, or in tea — all forms are effective. Getting ginger in any form into your system will help to settle your stomach. Ginger is my remedy of choice for stomach distress from flu, car or motion sickness, eating bad food, or poor food choices. I always carry a bottle of the tincture because it has so many other uses, such as warming me in frigid conference rooms and helping to fight a cold. While ginger is a very effective remedy, you may need frequent doses. It is not unusual to experience improvement within moments of taking the ginger and for your symptoms to return in 15–20 minutes. Just keep taking it.

The standard dose for the tincture is 1–2 droppersful, which can be taken every 15 minutes if necessary. Gnaw on fresh ginger root as needed, eating 1/4 teaspoon or more. The dose for capsules is 1–2 capsules and the dose for powdered herb is 1/4–1/2 teaspoon, which can be swallowed with water or may be emptied into water and drunk for more rapid effect. Or slice 1–3 teaspoons of fresh ginger into 2 cups of water and simmer for 10 minutes to make a lovely tea that will halt nausea and settle the stomach.

Have you noticed that ALL sushi restaurants serve pickled ginger? They do and for good reason! The Japanese and Chinese historically have used ginger as a primary antidote for "fish poison," meaning bad or tainted fish. (You would think that people who eat raw fish would suffer indigestion more often — perhaps they don't because they combine every bite of sushi with a slice of ginger.)

Speaking of sushi, *horseradish or wasabi* (a type of horseradish) also is an antidote for fish poison. (Isn't THAT interesting!) The Japanese traditionally serve horseradish with sushi, eastern European Jews traditionally serve horseradish with gefilte fish, and Americans serve horseradish with roast beef. Therapeutically, horseradish disperses stagnation. It keeps things moving and helps with digestion. While I don't carry horseradish with me, it is an excellent emergency medicine found in many homes, restaurants, and grocery stores. I recommend a teaspoon of grated horseradish — it is tasty on a cracker. One other great emergency use of horseradish is that it will enable you to urinate when you cannot. It also clears the sinuses and warms you when you feel chilled.

When I was growing up in New Jersey, many diners ("greasy spoons," my father called them) sold Tums and Pepto Bismol at the cash register. They knew that people needed help digesting that high fat, low fiber, and high salt food! Perhaps they needed some ginger or horseradish.

Fennel, a spice found in many kitchens, is a great remedy for indigestion. If you've ever been in an

INDIGESTION

Indian restaurant, you likely passed a bowl of fennel seeds at the front door. Many patrons take a pinch or small handful of fennel and chew them on the way home. Fennel, eaten as seeds or powdered, in capsules, brewed as tea, or taken in tincture form, clears gas and bloating. I have watched friends who were doubled over with the pain of acute gas resume normal activities within 20 minutes of taking fennel. Fennel tastes like licorice. It is a wonderful remedy for pregnant or nursing moms because it increases mothers' milk. In fact, fennel taken by a nursing mom is an excellent remedy for her nursing child with colic.

The Chinese have a patent remedy (a commercial herbal preparation that is sold over-the-counter) for indigestion called *Pills Curing* (also known as Kan Ning Wan or Pills Culing). Take 1 vial and repeat several hours later if necessary. This is available in Chinese herb shops and Oriental markets around the world. It also relieves constipation.

Have an ulcer type pain that feels hot? The herb *meadowsweet* helps with headaches and stomach pain. Take 1 dropperful, hourly or as needed. Or drink a tea made from 1 tablespoon of the dried herb steeped in 2 cups of recently boiled water. Drink $1/4 - 1/2$ cup every half hour.

Chamomile is THE herb of choice for indigestion linked to stress. Widely available in restaurants, grocery stores, and health food stores, chamomile is a well-known and tasty tea that contains no caffeine. Very mild, it is suitable for children, pregnant and nursing moms, and for people on a wide range of medications. Personally, I find that chamomile tea prepared from a single tea bag is only a pleasant beverage, not a remedy for indigestion. To settle your stomach, count on using no fewer than 4 tea bags or (even better) 2 tablespoons of dried chamomile herb for 1 cup of water. I carry the 1 ounce tincture for travel — 1 dropperful does the trick and makes a tasty "instant" tea.

Chamomile tincture is a very fast, very effective remedy. On a recent camping trip with a friend and her 4-year-old daughter, the daughter got into the marshmallows before lunch of our last day. We had been planning to hike out that afternoon. Well, little Emily was holding her stomach and wasn't going ANYWHERE. We gave her 2 drops of chamomile tincture and repeated the dose every 20 minutes. (Feeling stressed, I personally took a dropperful.) Emily stopped holding her stomach and visibly relaxed. (I felt less stressed.) About an hour later, we had packed our tents and were on our way. We offered Emily more, but she said her tummy was fine. Success! For adults: 1–2 dropperful, every half hour until symptoms clear.

Try *bitters* for indigestion. Bitters refers to a

INDIGESTION

variety of herbs or herbal combinations that taste bitter, stimulate digestion, and clear indigestion. Many herbalists make their own bitters combinations, with herbs that may include gentian, dandelion root, yarrow, and yellow dock. (You can make a GREAT combination from 10 parts gentian root, 4 parts bitter orange peel, and 1 part cardamom. Powder, place in a bottle or bag, and label. Take 1/4–1/2 teaspoon doses before meals or 1/4 teaspoon doses every 15 minutes to clear indigestion — stir into water and drink.) A ready-made version is *Swedish Bitters*, found in health food stores.

Umeboshi plum or umeboshi paste is a food that settles indigestion. Found in natural food stores in the macrobiotics section, this condiment is widely available in Japanese kitchens. Be prepared for the very salty taste. Take half teaspoon doses, hourly or until symptoms clear. Umeboshi has another, remarkable use: It will stop you or a child from crying — try it!

One holistic physician highly recommends *digestive enzymes* for indigestion. Open 1–2 capsules of digestive enzymes, add to a quarter cup of water, and drink. Do you have any *probiotics*, with names such as acidophilus, bifidus, and others? Take 1–2 capsules hourly until indigestion subsides.

Homeopathic Remedies

Acidil and *Nux vomica 30c* — described at the beginning of this chapter — provide relief from many forms of indigestion. As I type this section, I have Acidil in my pocket! I recommend *Arsenicum 30c* as the best general remedy for food poisoning. I also think of it anytime someone has bad stomach pain or indigestion with vomiting. Take 1 Acidil or 1–3 Nux vomica or Arsenicum pellets every 15 minutes until symptoms pass. (See the section on "Homeopathic Remedies" in the chapter on Diarrhea for additional suggestions.)

Indigestion in the Wilderness

Charcoal often clears indigestion. (See the section on Diarrhea in the Wilderness.) Additional wilderness remedies for indigestion include the tea prepared from the *inner bark of black (sweet) or yellow birch trees.* To prepare the bark, prune a small branch from the tree, strip off the outer bark and then the inner bark. Simmer 1 tablespoon of the inner bark in 2 cups of water for 20 minutes. Drink half a cup of tea every 30 minutes. Chew on a small twig while you are waiting for the tea — it tastes like wintergreen.

In the southeastern United States, you can drink a tea made from *kudzu root.* Simmer 2 tablespoons of cleaned and cut-up root in 2 cups of water for 20 minutes. Drink half a cup of tea every 30 minutes. It clears indigestion and diarrhea.

Indigestion Summary of Remedies

General recommendations:

- Breathe.
- Take time for yourself.
- Fast for 12–24 hours.
- Eat lightly: Light broths, tea and toast, crackers.
- Avoid fried and high fat foods.

Herbal and food remedies:

- Ginger.
- Horseradish.
- Fennel seed.
- Chamomile tincture.
- Umeboshi plum.
- Bitters.
- Chinese: Pills Curing.

Homeopathic remedies:

- Acidil or Nux vomica 30c.

Essential oils:

- Peppermint essential oil.

Supplements:

- Activated charcoal.
- Probiotics.
- Food enzymes.

Top packable remedies:

- Acidil or Nux vomica.
- Peppermint essential oil.
- Ginger candy, ginger capsules, or ginger tincture.
- Activated charcoal.

Top wilderness remedies:

- Charcoal (not the kind for grilling!).
- Black (sweet) or yellow birch inner bark or twigs.
- Kudzu root.

INSOMNIA

At the lecture, you couldn't keep your eyes open. Now, back at your hotel room, you can't fall asleep. Tomorrow is your big presentation — you need to be at your best, you finally have gone to bed, and you are wide awake. Or you are exhausted from traveling, lie down in bed, find yourself shaking and utterly unable to sleep.

Many of us are sensitive when it comes to sleep. We handle so many stresses in our lives, we accomplish so much, do so many things. But interfere with our sleep and our happiness, productivity, and sense of well-being disappear. We are more prone to colds and flu when our sleep is below par. Our endurance, strength, and focus diminish. We feel rotten!

Eliminate Stimulants

So what can we do? Begin reducing or eliminating those things that awaken or stress you during the evening.

Avoid caffeine in beverages. Foods that awaken you include all caffeine products: This means no coffee or tea with dinner. Caffeine sensitive people may need to eliminate caffeine after 12 noon! (By the way, decaffeinated teas and coffee still have caffeine — just less of it.) Green tea has caffeine. Many so-called herbal blend teas have caffeine; if the tea contains black tea or green tea, it has caffeine. Chamomile and mint teas, or teas with names like Sleepy Time or Nighty Night typically have no caffeine. Many soft drinks contain caffeine, especially colas, Mountain Dew, Surge, and Jolt! Read labels.

Avoid taking drugs that contain caffeine. Examine the labels of any drugs, especially over-the-counter-drugs, to see if they contain caffeine. Drugs that commonly include caffeine are decongestants, weight loss products, painkillers, and products to relieve cramps, among others. Often, the amount of caffeine in 1 dose is equivalent to the caffeine in a cup of coffee! If you need a decongestant to sleep and your decongestant contains caffeine, it won't help you sleep. Many medications are available without caffeine — you may wish to ask your pharmacist. Also, be alert to the presence of ma huang or ephedra in your travel pharmacy; these products may work well but easily can keep you awake. Pseudoephedrine, a pharmaceutical decongestant found in Sudafed and a number of other medications, can keep you awake. Read the label.

Avoid foods that keep you awake. The one piece of chocolate may not bother you, but that glorious "Death by Chocolate" dessert you ate at 11 p.m. may keep you awake for hours. Many people find that heavy or fatty foods such as barbecued ribs, goose, or pastries keep them awake.

Certain liquors will keep you awake. Red wine keeps many people wide awake, white wine awakens fewer people. Also, be alert to liquors that put you to sleep but result in troubled sleep. Abstinence, reduced consumption, or a change to "cleaner" beverages such as vodka may help.

Eat Earlier to Improve Your Sleep

Eating late keeps many travelers awake. While traveling, there are so many things to do that we often are pulled far from our accustomed schedules. Instead of your accustomed 6 or 7 p.m. dinner, you may be eating at 9 or 10. How late you finish eating makes a big difference in how you sleep. If you are suffering from insomnia and are eating several hours later than your accustomed time, try eating earlier.

Increasing the foods that aid relaxation can assist with your sleep. As a rule, high carbohydrate foods are more sedating than protein or fat. Many healthy travelers carefully limit their consumption of carbohydrates during the day for energy or weight loss reasons. Evening is the time to have a baked potato, rice, beans, or any other high carbohydrate food. If you are going to eat a piece of bread today, have it with dinner.

Consuming foods high in tryptophan can help you sleep. In the United States, who can forget eating turkey at Thanksgiving and then watching or experiencing the stupor? That stupor comes partly from overeating and partly from the turkey, which is high in tryptophan. Other foods that are high in tryptophan include tuna, milk and yogurt, bananas, dates, figs, whole grains, and nut butters. Remember that glass of warm milk at bedtime? It can help you sleep. (But brush your teeth before going to sleep!)

Quiet Time

Too much excitement experienced too late in the day can keep us awake. Have you gone to a late night concert, performed in a late sporting event, watched an emotional movie, or simply seen the late night news? What were you doing, what were you thinking, within two hours of your proposed bed-time? If you were excited and it was late, sheer excitement can keep you awake. In this case, you want to *find a way to wind down* or schedule your fun earlier. (Yeah, right!) Deep breathing, slow repetitive movements, prayer or meditation, writing, or a warm bath may help.

Breathe

Deep breathing just before bed is one of my favorite remedies for insomnia. It is cheap (free!), can be done anywhere, and takes very little effort or planning. Preferably, do this before you lie down,

INSOMNIA

perhaps in a chair, after you have completed all preparations for bed. Close your eyes, relax your body, and breathe in all the way down to your navel. Slowly exhale. Imagine breathing in calm and peace, imagine breathing out stress and anxiety. Maintain your deep breathing and your visualization for at least 5 minutes. Slowly open your eyes. Slip into bed, continuing to think of calm and peace. ZZZZZZZZZ.

Light, Dark, and Noise

Ever try to sleep with the lights on? Some people can, some people can't. Regardless, most people find that they fall asleep more easily in total darkness than at other times. When staying in hotels, I look forward to the total darkness provided by the blackout curtains that many hotels use. I sleep SO well that I often leave vowing to hang similar curtains at home! Total darkness sends a strong message to our brain that it REALLY is time to sleep. Total darkness also gives the pineal gland a time for rest and restoration, making sleep far more restful.

To increase the darkness for sleep, obtain a *sleep mask*. (You won't always be in the perfect hotel room.) Travel stores carry sleep masks, some airlines give them away on overseas flights, and you also may find them in drugstores. Some people swear by sleep masks containing magnets, such as the sleep mask manufactured by Nikken (a multi-level marketing company based in Japan), finding that use of the mask is calming and greatly enhances sleep.

Does noise keep you awake? Living in North Georgia, I have grown accustomed to sleeping in complete silence. When traveling, additional sound keeps me awake. I take charge of my environment by carrying a pair of foam *earplugs*. They are found in travel stores, drugstores, and hardware stores; they are inexpensive and work extremely well. If lack of sound keeps you awake, consider carrying a low-weight radio or cassette, CD, or white noise player with earplugs. These are widely available in specialty electronics stores such as Radio Shack or The Sharper Image, in drugstores, and in department stores.

Exercise

Have you ever traveled and just ached from the lack of exercise? Sometimes, your failure to fall asleep is linked to your lack of physical activity. Sitting on a plane for 20 hours, sitting in a conference, attending a workshop, driving in a car all day — these activities may exhaust you but do not provide exercise. Many of us need a minimum level of *exercise* in order to sleep. Taking a long walk, going for a run, swimming, or engaging in your sport on a daily basis may be enough to ensure a good night's sleep. Try to exercise at least two hours before bed because exercise can awaken you. In fact, a walk is a great choice during the afternoon break at conferences — skip the coffee and take a walk!

Baths

How about a *warm bath*? For some people, this is the only thing they need to promote good, quality sleep while on the road. Adding 10 drops of *lavender essential oil* to about a tablespoon of milk or shampoo and stirring this into the bath makes the bath more calming and gives you an aromatic and spa-like experience. (A shower does NOT have the same effect!) Plan on spending at least 10–20 minutes in the bath to gain the full, sleep inducing effect. Afterwards, place a few drops of lavender essential oil on your pillow, pajamas, or wrist to help you to relax and sleep. Ahhh.

Dehydration

Are you one of those people who falls asleep easily when traveling but then awakens in the middle of the night and has trouble falling back asleep? If this happens only when you travel, you may be dehydrated. Try drinking an additional 16–32 ounces of *water* each day. (But don't drink it just before bedtime!)

INSOMNIA

Herbal Remedies

In my opinion, our choices of food, lifestyle, and environment are far more important to the quality of our sleep than herbs that we take as supplements. Still, herbs can be invaluable at promoting good quality sleep. Sometimes, you just need more help. I ALWAYS carry sleep herbs when I travel.

If you can fall asleep but cannot stay asleep even when you are home, you may be fluid (yin) deficient. Try drinking more water. If that doesn't work, try an herbal remedy. Have 1–3 cups of *marshmallow root tea* each day. Simmer 6 tea bags or 1 tablespoon of the cut-up herb in 4 cups of water for 10–20 minutes. Alternatively, take 1 dropperful of marshmallow root tincture 3 times per day. You will feel less dry and will sleep better. You can purchase the herbs at a natural food store. Marshmallow, which is a yin tonic, promotes sleep in yin deficient people. (Prepared) *rehmannia root* and *asparagus root*, both from the Chinese herbal tradition, are even more effective yin tonics. Simmer 1 ounce of rehmannia root or asparagus root in 4 cups of water for 10–20 minutes, and drink 1 cup 3 times per day.

For children, *chamomile* is my top choice for sleep. It is sweet, tasty, settles the stomach, and clears anxiety and can be drunk as a tea. It works for adults, too! Many children especially appreciate the glycerine-based tincture that comes in a dropper bottle. The brand Herbs for Kids makes a good product. Follow directions on the label. For adults, I recommend alcohol-based tinctures, which are stronger and keep longer than the glycerine. (Yes, chamomile tincture can work for you even if the tea doesn't affect you. The tincture is amazing!)

My personal favorite is *kava kava*. Kava commonly is used to clear anxiety and especially helps those of us who go to bed thinking. Kava has a surprising and unusual taste that many dislike but gladly endure because it works so well. Forget the capsules and the pills — get the tincture! Standard dose is 1–4 droppersful. Oh yes, worried about mixing kava with alcohol? You might have had a few drinks with dinner? The cautions on the bottle about not mixing alcohol and kava pertain to much higher doses of kava, not to the therapeutic dose to help you sleep.

Passion flower, *valerian*, and *hops*, used separately or (even better) together provide a strong, sleep inducing combination. Take 1–4 droppersful before bed. This combination is especially helpful for people who are easily excited. In high enough doses, valerian is a sedative. (It is not, by the way, related to the drug Valium.) **Caution: A very small percentage of people are sensitive to valerian and find it wakes them up!** If you have never used it, try a small dose before you travel. (If it wakes you up, use *skullcap* herb instead, 1–4 droppersful before bed.)

Ashwagandha, an Ayurvedic herb, is the herb of choice for people who tend towards exhaustion and insomnia. A client of mine, exhausted by her constant travel to tend to an ailing parent and feeling the stresses and strains of her own family responsibilities, asked for help. She described arriving home utterly exhausted and completely unable to sleep. Deep breathing, meditation, long walks — nothing seemed to help. She tried ashwagandha in powdered form, mixing 1 teaspoon into soy milk 3 times per day. Within days, she could sleep! Her sleep was deep and restful and she felt much less tired. Ashwagandha can be taken in capsules, in powdered form, or as a tincture, and all work well. One particularly good way to take ashwagandha is 1 teaspoon in scalded milk with honey. It has a unique taste, somewhat earthy and sweet.

I've got to warn you though. Ashwagandha, taken for more than 1 month, is an effective aphrodisiac! It really increases sex drive. Importantly, it increases sex drive — both in men and women — while nourishing the body. Michael Tierra, a prominent herbalist and the author of *The Way of Herbs*, describes ashwagandha as the "most potent" aphrodisiac. One physician friend who loved the energy enhancing and calming qualities of this herb abruptly stopped using it after 1 month — she found the aphrodisiac qualities to be way too strong!

Essential Oils

Lavender essential oil is soothing and relaxing. (See the previous section on "Baths.") Two or 3 drops on a handkerchief placed on your pillow or chest is a great sleep aid. Try it for airline travel.

Supplements

Melatonin is a great sleep aid, especially when travel has changed your sleep schedule or you are traveling across time zones. Take .5 milligrams just before going to sleep.

INSOMNIA

Insomnia Summary of Remedies

Lifestyle suggestions:

- No caffeine after noon (coffee, tea, drugs, soda, chocolate).
- Drink more water.
- Breathe.
- Meditate.
- Eat high carbohydrate foods in the evening.
- Eat high tryptophan foods.
- Finish eating early in the evening.
- Drink warm milk before bed.
- Take a warm bath (with lavender essential oil).
- Take 2 hours quiet time before bed.

Herbs:

- Marshmallow.
- Kava kava.
- Chamomile.
- Passion flower, hops, and valerian.
- Ashwagandha.

Essential oils:

- Lavender essential oil.

Supplements:

- Melatonin.

Other sleep aids:

- Eye mask.
- Earplugs.
- White noise or sound generator.

INSOMNIA

JET LAG

Jet lag is the physical and emotional discomfort we experience after rapidly passing through multiple time zones. People may experience headaches, lack of appetite, profound sleepiness, exhaustion, irritability, or disorientation. The effects of jet lag vary greatly from person to person, but the effects are very real. People experience jet lag in different ways and to different degrees.

Jet lag always has fascinated me. It only occurs with travel from east to west or west to east. When traveling across fewer than 12 time zones, traveling east is more likely to produce jet lag than traveling west. All people who travel by air across at least two time zones experience jet lag. Although some may not notice it and others may have debilitating symptoms, everyone "gets" it. It is a function of our time, that today we can move so quickly that our bodies literally are left behind.

Jet lag costs us time and money. For the vacationer, jet lag may ruin a substantial portion of a trip or may result in illness following the trip home. The person traveling for business will be at a competitive disadvantage in any negotiation immediately following rapid travel across time zones.

My first major experience with jet lag was after

flying to Australia. I thought I knew what to expect. I arrived in Sydney, 13 time zones from my home on the east coast of the United States. No headache, no malaise, no exhaustion. "I don't have jet lag," I said to myself. An hour later, I was walking along the beautiful Sydney Harbor looking at the blue skies and the fabulous skyline. Then, for no apparent reason, I burst into tears. I couldn't stop crying. I looked around — nothing was wrong, everything was fine. But I felt as though I was at the bottom of a dark and dank pit, completely lost and utterly incapable of continuing on my journey. Finally, I called friends in Canberra. They asked how my trip had gone, I snuffled on the phone, and my friend Helen exclaimed, "You have jet lag!" She, a seasoned traveler, assured me that it would pass and that I would not always feel this way. She was right. It took about 3 days.

Jet Lag Reduction Program

The heart of the jet lag reduction program is *rest*, *rehydration*, and *resetting your inner clock*. Judicious use of caffeine helps. Supplementation also helps.

At least 3 days prior to your trip, *stop drinking coffee* and all other sources of caffeine. Begin fully hydrating your body with high quality *water*, at least 1 ounce of water daily for every 2 pounds of body weight or, at a minimum, 64 ounces of pure water a day. Take at least 3,000 milligrams of natural *vitamin C* each of those 3 days. Obtain *Rescue Remedy*, a product for stress available at most health food stores, and begin taking 4 drops at least 3 times (preferably 6 times) per day. Rest a minimum of 8 hours per night.

Three days before your trip, *change your exposure to light*. When planning to travel east, avoid outdoor light for the last 3 hours of daylight, and go to bed earlier than usual. When planning to travel west, avoid outdoor light for the first 3 hours of daylight.

Take No Jet-Lag. This homeopathic combination addresses many jet lag symptoms before they arise. Chew 1 tablet of No Jet-Lag upon boarding the plane, 1 tablet every 2 hours of flight, and 1 tablet after landing. Then, take 1 tablet as needed for fatigue. This is a GREAT remedy — if I could only use 1 jet lag remedy, this would be it! (It contains Arnica 30c, Bellis perennis 30c, Chamomilla 30c, Ipecacuanha 30c, and Lycopodium 30c.) Some people find that it completely eliminates jet lag. Find it in health food stores or purchase it on the Internet. One caution: No Jet-Lag contains the sweetener sorbitol. If you are sorbitol sensitive, it can nauseate you.

To assist the pineal gland in resetting your

inner clock, some travelers take a small dose of *melatonin*, a natural hormone. Three days before your trip, take .5 milligrams at breakfast time. On the day of your trip take it at breakfast time for your destination. Melatonin also will help you to sleep. Take it just before going to sleep.

Prepare a *travel bag* with everything you need for your trip. Pack at least 1–2 liters of pure *water* for times when beverage service is not available. Obtain a soft and comfortable *sleep mask* and noise-reduction *earplugs*, both available at travel stores. At your local health food store, obtain *vitamin C*, preferably a natural C with 1,000 milligrams per dose. (I like traveling with Emer'gen-C, an excellent and tasty product in individual packs that dissolve in water.) Pack any herbs that you have used to assist you in falling asleep; good choices include *kava kava*, a *passion flower-hops-valerian* combination, or *chamomile*. If you have never used sleep herbs, I recommend that you begin with a 1 ounce bottle of chamomile tincture. Obtain a 1 ounce bottle of *Siberian ginseng* tincture, available at your health food store. If you choose to use melatonin, purchase .5 milligram doses at your local health food store or pharmacy. Pack 3 or more high quality *protein or meal replacement bars*. (My favorites are Balance Bars and Boulder Bars.) Pack *candied ginger* to eat if you feel a cold coming on, if you become chilled, if you feel nauseated, or if you begin to feel motion sickness. If you will be traveling for three or more night-time hours, pack *socks* for sleeping or extra soft slippers. Be sure to pack your *toothbrush and toothpaste*. Try to finish preparing your travel bag at least three days prior to your trip.

Carry your travel bag with you.

Once you have boarded the plane and settled yourself in your seat, chew 1 No Jet-Lag tablet. Look at your watch — plan to take 1 tablet every 2 hours and upon arrival. Breathe. Relax.

As soon as the plane departs, set your watch to the current time at your destination. Note the time and begin thinking in terms of the new time. From now on, be disciplined and think only of the destination time. Remember, you are resetting your inner clock, not just your watch. While you are awake, check your watch at least every hour, telling yourself the time and what you ordinarily do at that time.

Upon takeoff, drink no less than 16 ounces of water. Drink only bottled water. You have no idea of the source of the plane's water or the cleanliness of the water storage. Talk the steward into letting you have a large or multiple small bottles of water to keep at your seat. Drink 8 ounces of water for every hour that you are on the plane.

Take 1 gram (1,000 milligrams) of vitamin C. Take NO ALCOHOL and NO CAFFEINE. No caffeine means no coffee, no tea, no colas, no Mountain Dew, no Surge, no Jolt, and no chocolate. (OK, maybe just a little chocolate!) No alcohol means no liquor, no cordials, no beer, and no wine. If you feel bad about missing free drinks on international flights, just tell yourself that both caffeine and alcohol are dehydrating and that dehydration makes jet lag much worse. Feel virtuous in your discipline.

Try taking adaptogens, herbs that assist the body in adapting to change. An herbal combination that will help with jet lag consists of *astragalus, schizandra, and Siberian ginseng*. People who commonly experience nausea, motion sickness, or other digestive problems could add *ginger*. This combination strongly enhances the immune system, helps to stop what the Chinese call the "leakage of qi" (loss of energy), builds energy, and improves rest times. It is a warming formula that may be too "hot" for people who usually feel hot when everyone else is cold. For hot people, I recommend a combination of *astragalus and burdock root*. Single adaptogenic herbs include *ashwagandha*, astragalus, burdock root, *American ginseng*, *panax ginseng*, schizandra, Siberian ginseng, *suma*, and *tienchi ginseng*. Common dosages are 1–4 droppersful or 0.5 to 2.0 milliliters, or 2 capsules, 1–3 times per day.

Try taking demulcent herbs that moisten from

the inside out if you get stuffy when you fly. Take *marshmallow root* or *asparagus root*, either 2 capsules, 1 dropperful of the tincture, or 1 cup of the tea every hour or two. These demulsifying (softening and moistening) herbs soothe the mucus membranes that become irritated by the dry cabin air. The membranes will relax and the stuffiness will disappear. Spraying your face with water or a saline solution also will help. Keep drinking your water!

Plan to go to sleep at your regular sleep time according to your watch. This may be very different from the schedule on the plane. As you approach "bedtime" begin winding down. Do as much of your sleep preparation routine as you can. *Take your relaxing herbs* (chamomile, kava kava, or passion flower-valerian-hops) and melatonin, take off your shoes, and put on your slippers. Finally, put in your earplugs, turn off your seat light, place your seat in its reclining position, put on your sleep mask, and begin slowing and deepening your breathing. The darkness provided by your sleep mask is key to resetting your inner clock. *Believe that you will fall asleep.* Even if you do not immediately fall asleep, continue to rest in this position. Try your best to sleep or rest for at least four hours. (Do not worry that you will insult the staff or look stupid.)

Avoid all light until dawn at your destination. At dawn, feel free to look deeply at light. Watching the sunrise will really help! Drink at least another 16 ounces of water and take 1 gram of vitamin C.

Today, what you eat, drink, and think will make a huge difference in how you fare during the next 24 hours. Look at your watch and consciously tell yourself the destination time. ("I am in Japan, it is 8 a.m., it is time for breakfast.") Remember, you are anchoring yourself in the destination time.

At morning for your destination, drink 1–2 cups of *coffee*, *tea*, or *hot chocolate*. Go ahead and have the espresso! Yes, this is the time for caffeine. The caffeine helps your body to catch up to the new time zone. Also, if you regularly drink caffeine as a morning beverage, drinking it now helps to cement the mind set that this is indeed morning. You will NOT have any caffeine after noon. Absolutely NO caffeine at night! Remember, you still are resetting your inner clock.

When breakfast is served, DO NOT eat sugary pastries. *Try to avoid sweets*; they slow you down. If nothing at breakfast appeals to you, open your travel bag and eat 1 of your protein bars. Have another vitamin C and plan on taking at least 3 grams that day. The vitamin C helps to clear toxins from your system (including all the fumes you inhale on board a jet). Vitamin C also helps the immune system and provides a minor energy boost. After breakfast, have another 16 ounces of water.

After You Land

During the morning, *spend at least 15 minutes outdoors*, preferably with your face in the sunshine. Standing in the shade does not count! Sun on your face, even if obscured by clouds, nourishes the pineal gland and helps reset your inner clock. This is a great time to take a walk, which will relieve some of the stagnation of the long flight.

Before each eating event drink at least 16 ounces of pure water. Assume you still are dehydrated. This is your first day at your destination and you need to continue drinking your water. Many planes fly with only 5 percent humidity. The combination of low humidity and your (likely) lack of sleep will deplete your body fluids, also known as your yin. Drink between a half gallon and a full gallon of water that first day, the second day, and the third day.

Feel free to have a mid-morning snack, lunch, and a mid-afternoon snack but *plan on eating as lightly as possible*. Simply by traveling to another time zone, your digestive system has been stressed and fatigued. Taste rather than gorge. Choose low-fat foods and be gentle on your system. Avoid heavy sauces. Avoid deep fried foods. Do combine non-starchy vegetables (green leafy vegetables) with protein. Freely *take herbal digestive aids*, such as chamomile and ginger. Avoid starchy carbohydrates, like breads, cake, cookies, rice, and potatoes until dinnertime at your destination time. Why? They make you sleepy. Reserve them for when you are winding down.

Feeling tired? *Do NOT go back to sleep.* Going back to sleep would let you slip back to your departure time zone. Don't do it! Walk around, drink water, take deep breaths, read, exercise, see what other people are doing, strike up a conversation. Do ANYTHING to avoid sleep. By the way, this is a great time to have some *ginseng*! Two droppersful of ginseng tincture, 1 10 milliliter bottle of ginseng extract, 1–2 tea bags steeped for 5 minutes in hot water, or a teaspoon of the root simmered in three cups of water for an hour (serves 2–3 people) will help recharge your batteries. (If you have high blood pressure, don't take panax ginseng — choose American or Siberian ginseng instead.) A packet of Emer'gen-C dissolved in 8 ounces of water will lift your energy.

If possible, *avoid alcohol*. If you must have alcohol, limit your consumption to evening. Try to have as little as possible. Alcohol places great stress on the liver, which regulates many of the body's activities. You are consciously avoiding foods and beverages that depress body functions. On the other hand, alcohol can be relaxing — for people who drink, 1 drink in the evening may help you to sleep.

Sound like a lot to do? It is worth it. You'll see!

Jet Lag Summary

3 days before trip:

- Drink 64 ounces of water per day.
- Take 3,000 milligrams of natural vitamin C each day.
- Take 4 drops of Rescue Remedy at least 3 (preferably 6) times per day.
- No caffeine 3 days prior to trip (you'll have some after you arrive).
- Traveling east: avoid outdoor light for the last 3 hours of daylight.
- Traveling west: avoid outdoor light for the first 3 hours of daylight.
- Pack your travel bag with your supplements, water, sleep mask, and ear plugs.

Departure day:

- Set watch to destination time upon boarding plane.
- Chew 1 tablet of No Jet-Lag upon boarding plane, 1 tablet every 2 hours of flight, and 1 tablet after landing.
- Drink 8 ounces of water for every hour on the plane and at least 64 ounces per day for the first 3 days at your destination.
- No alcohol. No sugar.
- If you tend to get airsick, take ginger every 15–60 minutes.
- Eat lightly.

Arrival day:

- Feel free to have caffeine at breakfast time for your destination.
- Eat a no sugar, low carbohydrate breakfast.
- Natural light, outdoors if possible, at destination.
- Walk or other exercise.
- Do not nap at destination.
- Enjoy a high carbohydrate, low-fat dinner.
- Go to bed early.

Top packable remedies:

- Sleep mask.
- Earplugs.
- Socks or soft slippers.
- Vitamin C.
- Kava kava.
- Siberian ginseng.
- Ginger.
- No Jet-Lag.
- Bottled water.
- Protein bars.

MISSING MEDICINES

"I'm sure I brought my medication with me. I have my list, I checked it off. I know that it has to be somewhere." Turning to your husband/wife/travel companion, you ask, "Have you seen my meds?" No, you are told, look in your suitcase. Of course, by now, you have turned your suitcase over on the bed, or you have dumped your pack out on the floor of the tent. You have made a mess, and you STILL have no medication.

You begin going through all your pockets. You wonder when you last took your medication. Did you leave it in the last restaurant? By now, you have been feeling foolish for at least the last half hour, and you are beginning to worry. You NEED that medication. You NEED whatever it is that you have left behind.

What are you going to do? Well, if you are in the woods, you have the choice of doing without, borrowing from a companion, finding whatever you need in the wild (you remembered to bring your Peterson Field Guide, didn't you?), calling for help on your satellite phone, or turning back. If you are in an urban area, you can tell yourself that things could be worse. At least you are not lost in the woods!

Planning for Possible Loss of Your Medications, Herbs, and Supplements

No matter how careful you are, you can forget things, bags can be stolen, and accidents can happen. I recommend that all travelers *carry photocopies of their prescriptions* with them, just in case they lose or forget their medication. Be sure that your prescription includes the name and amount of the medication, the name and phone number of the pharmacy, and the name and phone number of the prescribing doctor. You may need to add some of this information yourself.

Pack all medication, herbs, and supplements in your carry-on or hand luggage. Airlines misplace luggage. Trains misplace luggage. Buses misplace luggage. Stuff gets stolen. Keep your medication, herbs, and supplements close to you.

Make a master list of all medications that you take, where you obtain them, and why you take those medications. Do you take a baby aspirin daily to reduce the threat of stroke? Do you take valerian to help you to sleep? Do you carry echinacea in case you feel a cold coming on? What about your daily vitamin? Your vitamin C? Whatever you use, add it to your master list, including where you obtain it and why you take it.

If you take a commercial (prepackaged) herbal combination, note all names of the combination listed on the product (many Chinese patent medicines, which have both a marketing name and a traditional name, are available around the world), the manufacturer or preparing herbalist, and when possible, the list of the herbs in the product. When possible, make a photocopy of the packaging. Whatever you use, add it to your master list, including where you obtain it and why you take it.

If you take a personalized herbal formula, list the names of all the herbs in your native language and in Latin. If the herb is Chinese (or any other non-western tradition), try to list the herbs in your language, in the herbalist's language, and in Chinese. Your herbalist can best guide you with this task, and may direct you to a good herbal text.

For pharmaceuticals, go to your local pharmacy and find out the store's policy for refilling and shipping prescriptions. Confirm that the pharmacy can refill your prescriptions on your request and confirm that the pharmacy can ship to you based upon your phone order. If a more current prescription is needed, contact your physician for a renewed prescription and place the renewed prescription with your pharmacy. If your pharmacy does not provide shipping, contact one that does. An increasing number of pharmacies that make their living by shipping can be found on the Internet. Add the pharmacy's phone and fax number to your master list.

For herbs and supplements, go to your preferred health food store and confirm that the store will ship to you based upon a phone order. Add the health food store's phone number and fax number to your master list.

Obtain a prepaid phone card. At the time of this writing, large discount warehouse stores provide some of the lowest prices in the United States and phone companies provide some of the highest! A prepaid card can save you a lot of money — hotels and public phones may charge hundreds of times the rate you would pay on a prepaid card. Obtain an international card for international travel. Check current prices and purchase a card.

Carry your master list in two places — with you in your pocket, purse, fanny pack, small personal luggage, or with your passport AND someplace else, such as in your luggage or backpack. Be sure to include all prescription and over-the-counter medications, herbs, homeopathics, and supplements (with attachments). If you know what you lost, you often can replace it. Depending upon where you are traveling, you may be able to replace all you have lost in local pharmacies, stores, and herb shops or by having something shipped. Your list will be invaluable.

Replacing Lost Medications, Herbs, and Supplements

Know that you can replace anything you have lost. (Personally, I start walking around looking for local plants. But that is me!)

Obtain a signed police, airline, or hotel manager's report detailing the time, date, and loss. If the police, airline, or manager do not ordinarily write such reports, you may write one of your own, signed both by you and the officer or a manager. If no official will sign, try to have someone else, even a travel companion, sign as a witness. You may need this later, especially if you will be replacing prescription drugs. It also may be helpful for insurance purposes.

Review your master list and determine what you need to replace. In metropolitan areas of the United States, you often can obtain everything you need in a large grocery that includes a pharmacy. In many other places, you may need to visit a pharmacy, natural products store, grocery, and herb shop. Phone books are helpful for obtaining the names and locations of the stores.

Replace prescription medicines FIRST. This often is the most difficult and time-consuming. Ask to see the pharmacist, show her or him your prescription copies, and ask for help. Charm and sincerity go a long way here. Local laws may be very strict — you may be asking a BIG favor of the pharmacist in requesting that she or he fill the prescription. If you can't fill your prescriptions locally, call your pharmacist and have them shipped. Many pharmacies will ship product to you almost anywhere in the world.

Having trouble obtaining replacement herbs and supplements? Consider having things shipped. (See the section above, "Planning for Possible Loss of Your Medication, Herbs, and Supplements.") This often is the least costly, least troublesome solution. The larger health food stores in my area ship all over the United States and occasionally around the world. Most professional herbalists keep meticulous records of your herbal combinations — some of them will ship directly to you. Know that UPS (United Parcel Service) and FedEx (Federal Express) ship to most places around the globe, often overnight.

Missing Medicines Summary

Planning for possible loss of medications, herbs, and supplements:

- Photocopy all prescriptions.
- Make a master list. Include what you take, why you take it, Latin or trade name, and phone and fax number of store that will refill or replace item. Confirm that stores will refill or replace from a phone call. Update all prescriptions as needed.
- Obtain a prepaid phone card.
- Carry your master list in 2 places.
- Carry your medications, herbs, and supplements with you.

Replacing lost medications, herbs, and supplements:

- Know you can replace everything.
- Obtain a signed report describing the loss.
- Review your master list.
- Replace prescription medications first. If you cannot replace items locally, have the items shipped to you.
- Replace all other medications, herbs, and supplements. If you cannot replace items locally, have the items shipped to you.

MISSING MEDICINES

MOTION SICKNESS

The day I finished writing this section, I closed my computer and drove to my martial arts class. Our instructor laid out mats and had us perform forward rolls — over and over again.

Although this is an important skill, it is not one that we usually practice, so it was an unaccustomed movement for me. We rolled continuously for around 30 minutes. At the end of class, my stomach hurt and I felt feverish and generally rotten. I mentioned to a classmate that I thought that I was getting sick, that it felt like flu. She considered a moment and said that maybe the rolling motion made me sick. Motion sickness!

I ran to the local grocery, went to the produce department, and broke off a small piece of ginger. I skinned it with my thumb and gnawed off a piece the size of the nail on my pinky. I chewed it and considered how I felt. No effect. I thought, "Well, I might as well pick up some water." By the time I reached the water, maybe 2 minutes later, I realized things had changed. No stomach ache. No fever. No nausea. Wow, I thought, gone in 2 minutes! Not quite. It started coming back. I chewed a little more, same result. Nausea gone for 5 minutes, nausea returns, chew more ginger, nausea gone for 5 minutes, chew more ginger. In all, I probably had 5 or 6 bites. Afterwards, I had dinner. Success!

The ginger, taken in raw form, relieved about 90 percent of my discomfort. Continued small doses proved important to my recovery. The raw ginger, taken in tiny bites, was mild enough to chew. Relief was almost immediate, but total recovery took some time. I did not feel the need to seek an additional remedy and was able to continue my activities. I definitely include raw ginger on the list of motion sickness remedies.

What Is Motion Sickness?

Motion sickness results when you experience a conflict between what you see and what you feel with the delicate mechanisms of your inner ear. It also results when your body cannot adjust to the unaccustomed change in what it perceives as vertical. People commonly experience motion sickness on boats, in cars, on planes, and in computer generated "virtual reality."

Herbal Remedies

My favorite all-time remedy for motion sickness is *ginger*. Ginger candy. Ginger tea. Ginger tincture. Ginger capsules. If it has real ginger in it, it will work. I highly recommend that people prone to motion sickness carry ginger on all trips.

You can find candied ginger in Oriental food markets (the lowest price source), in natural food markets, and in gourmet shops. The candy does not need refrigeration and packs well. Taste it before you go — some ginger is VERY sharp and may not be to your taste.

Ginger tea is available in Oriental food markets, natural food stores, and occasionally in grocery stores. You can make your own tea from fresh ginger, which is widely available in produce departments. Grate or slice approximately 1–2 inches of the root into 2 cups of water. Simmer for 20–30 minutes and drink. Personally, I find that the fresh ginger tea works best of all. You also can make the tea from ginger powder, which you can find in the spice department in groceries or in Oriental markets. Simmer 1 teaspoon of ginger powder in 2 cups of water for 20–30 minutes.

You can obtain ginger capsules at natural food and health stores. (These are just powdered ginger — the ground spice — that has been placed in capsules.) Many travelers bring a few capsules with them for emergencies. This is a very convenient form and, of course, requires no cooking and involves no fluids that could spill.

When I travel, I bring a 1 ounce bottle of ginger

tincture with me. When I feel distress, I take 1 drop-perful of the tincture. Advantages of the tincture include its easy packability and its immediate effect. In alcohol, the herb enters the bloodstream more quickly, so it works very fast. You can add 1–2 droppersful of ginger tincture to hot water for a quick and easy cup of tea on the road. Yum!

Ginger is SUCH a good remedy that I recommend ALL travelers take it with them. It is good for so many digestive problems, including nausea, gas, fish or other food poisoning, and many different stomach aches. It helps to clear a cold or flu before it takes hold and helps with cold and flu symptoms. It will warm you if you have become overly chilled. Soaking your feet in ginger tea will relieve foot aches from too much walking. Taken internally, it helps to relieve women's menstrual cramps. It is a delicious beverage that is mildly energizing but will not keep you awake. What a pal!

Begin any herbal motion sickness remedy at least 1 hour before travel. If taking ginger, take some every 15–60 minutes and more frequently when necessary. Although all forms of ginger are effective, I personally like the convenience and chewing of crystallized ginger.

Other herbal remedies for nausea include *peppermint* and *chamomile*. I find them much less effective than ginger, but use what you have.

Homeopathic Remedies

Travelers who prefer homeopathic remedies should try *Nux vomica 30c* or *Cocculus 30c*. Place 1–3 of the tiny pellets beneath your tongue about 1 hour prior to travel. Repeat this dose every 15 minutes, especially if you feel motion sickness. Other great choices include *Tabacum 10x* for people who get nauseated with headache and sometimes dizziness or *Petroleum 10x* for people who get nauseous with dizziness, heartburn, and possible belching. Use the same dose and frequency listed above. See "Choosing Homeopathic Remedies," page 12.

Food and Supplements

Eat lightly prior to travel and avoid acid foods like orange juice and coffee and fatty and fried foods. If travel also makes you nervous, take *Rescue Remedy*. *Vitamin B-6*, 100 mg. per day, helps some people to avoid nausea. Alternatively, eat at least 1 cup of *parsley* or *dark green leafy vegetables* per day. This food remedy helps some people avoid nausea.

Pharmaceutical Remedies

Medical doctors commonly recommend *Dramamine* (dimenhydrinate) for motion sickness. It has a long history of successful usage but many people do not like the common side effect — sleepiness. Review all contraindications prior to purchase. Dramamine cannot be taken with certain medications and should not be taken by people with glaucoma, enlarged prostate, emphysema, or chronic bronchitis. Do not take with alcohol. If you will be scuba diving, find another remedy because Dramamine can cause inebriation with high pressure. If you choose to take this medication, take it at least 1 hour prior to travel, and then every 4–6 hours.

More recent to the market is *Bonine* (meclizine). Many people prefer it to Dramamine because it doesn't make them as sleepy. If you choose to take this medication, take it at least 1 hour prior to travel, and then every 24 hours. Side effects include sleepiness, dry mouth, and possibly blurred vision.

Other people use a prescription skin patch called a *Transderm Scop*, which contains the drug scopolamine and must be applied 6–8 hours prior to travel. Apply the patch in the hairless area behind one ear. If you need assistance with motion sickness for more than 3 days, discard and replace the patch every 3 days, using alternate ears. Wash your hands thoroughly after touching the patch! Scopolamine may cause sleepiness, dry eyes, dry mouth, and a variety of other side effects. Consult the *Physicians' Desk Reference (PDR)* or *The People's Pharmacy* for further information.

Acupressure

You can use acupressure on yourself to eliminate motion sickness — you press and "grind" your thumb against the inside of your opposite wrist. Find the spot by following the base of your thumb two finger-widths below the "break" in your wrist. Feel the hollow spot? That's it! Called "Pericardium 6," "*P-6*," "Inner Gate," or "Neiguan," it is used for many different functions, including treatment of nausea, vomiting, digestive pain, acid reflux, hiccups, and belching. It also helps to sedate PMS emotionality and is generally calming to both men and women. This really works!

Natural products manufacturers have seized upon the proven value of this acupressure point and have provided a variety of *wrist bands and wrist straps* that stimulate P-6 for you. Available in natural products stores and from some health care professionals, these typically have a small plastic or magnetic bump that is placed directly over the point. The wrist bands and wrist straps cost $10–20. Both the plastic and magnetic versions have been found to be effective.

I recommend that motion sickness sufferers try these products and that they use them with ginger. They are a MUST for long sailing trips, even for individuals who have not yet suffered from motion sickness. Prolonged rough seas can do in anyone, but motion sickness doesn't have to happen to you.

Other Helpful Hints

When in a moving car, train, or ship, *focus your eyes on the horizon*. This will limit the movement that is disturbing you. If you tend towards motion sickness, *avoid reading*. Position yourself to minimize motion — on a plane, sit over the wing; in a car, sit in the front seat. When traveling by car, you may want to drive; many people experience less motion sickness when they drive than when they ride as passengers.

Many people are sensitive to the rocking motion on board boats and ships. Strive to *maintain your head in a perfectly vertical position*. When the ship rolls to the right, compensate by shifting to the left. *Fresh air* and well-ventilated spaces help many people. Move away and stay away from strong smells such as fish, diesel fumes, chemicals, or cooking smells.

Motion Sickness Summary of Remedies

Food recommendations:
- Eat lightly.
- Avoid coffee, orange juice, and fatty foods.

Herbal remedy:
- Ginger.

Homeopathic remedies:
- Nux vomica 30c.
- Cocculus 30c.
- Tabacum 10x.
- Petroleum 10x.

Supplements:
- Vitamin B-6.

Flower essences:
- Rescue Remedy.

Pharmaceutical remedies:
- Dramamine *or*
- Bonine *or*
- Scopolamine patch.

Acupressure:
- Press P-6 on both wrists.

Other helpful hints:
- Don't read.
- Gaze at the horizon.
- Hold head vertically.

Top packable remedies:
- Ginger in all forms.
- Nux vomica 30c.
- Motion sickness wrist straps.

MOTION SICKNESS

PARASITES

I had just come back from a great trip to Arizona and was sitting with my herbal study group. I was excited and ready to describe my trip. I felt flushed — was it the excitement? I found myself sweating — had it been that hard to bring my books into our study room? My abdomen hurt — was I starting my menses early with the stress of travel? I had a slight headache — dehydration from the plane? It was becoming increasingly hard to focus. My abdomen felt hot and the pain increased. I felt nauseated. I had diarrhea. Was it appendicitis? I was having trouble focusing. My colleagues, all medically trained, asked if I was OK. Oh, sure, I said, wondering how I would drive myself home. Wisely, my group insisted that a medical doctor check me for possible appendicitis.

Thirty minutes later, my doctor manually checked my appendix — no problem. She looked at me: still sweating, heart racing, nauseated, and in pain. She had one question for me: Had I been traveling? Yes, but it was all within the United States. No camping. No lake or river water. She laughed and said that if someone with my symptoms answered yes to travel, ANYWHERE, she treated the person for parasites. Why, I asked? She shrugged her shoulders, said that testing took too long, and treatment for parasites usually cleared the problem.

My doctor wrote out a prescription for a strong anti-parasite drug, Flagyl, which has common side effects of nausea, loss of appetite, and low energy. She told me that it was a "rough" but effective medicine and said that I had 48 hours to clear the symptoms on my own before filling the prescription. I began taking anti-parasite herbs, a combination of *black walnut hull*, *cascara sagrada*, *clove*, and *wormwood* every 20 minutes, and my symptoms shifted within an hour. Amazing! My condition changed so quickly that I wondered what really had happened. And I wondered how we get parasites and how many of us have them.

Who Has Parasites?

First of all, *everyone gets and has parasites*. Everyone. This includes rich and poor and people in rural, suburban, and metropolitan areas. People with pets and people without them. Outdoor types and office workers. One naturopathic doctor said that to be human means having parasites.

You believe you are different? You bathe every day, drink only bottled water, and eat only the cleanest food? Well, I suggest that you look at your skin under a 200x to 500x powered microscope. Those creatures you see moving on your skin may look as though they are from another planet. They are on you, they live on and in you, and they are called parasites. No amount of scrubbing will totally eliminate them. We probably need them! (Well, some of them.)

We get parasites from the air that we breathe, the surfaces that we touch, the water that we drink, and the food that we eat. Parasites are easily spread through human and animal contact, through feces, through raw foods, through sewage, through dirt, and by insects. Parasites are spread through simple handshakes, children's play, and sex. Really, the list goes on and on.

Parasites are living creatures that live on or in us, at our expense. They vary in size from the tiniest microorganisms visible only under high powered microscopes to worms measured in feet or meters. Most of the time, we live in balance with our parasites. Travel may introduce us to unaccustomed parasites that precipitate a major response in our bodies, making us ill.

Symptoms of parasite infestation may include dysentery, vomiting, profuse sweating, and many other uncomfortable symptoms. Minor symptoms include anal or ear itching, diarrhea, cravings for unusual foods (such as charcoal, dirt, clay, and raw rice), and major changes in appetite. Other symptoms include digestive disorders, many skin conditions, mental fog, memory problems, sleep problems, and various aches and pains.

Most travelers don't have time for testing. As my doctor suggested, *when you suspect parasites, treat for parasites*. My personal rule of thumb — assume parasites if the person has ear, nose, or anal itching. When traveling in areas of known contamination, assume you will come in contact with parasites (yes, even at five-star hotels) and respond accordingly. If non-sterile water touches your lips or eyes in those areas — you have parasites. Take immediate action.

Reducing the Likelihood of Parasite Infestation

You can reduce the likelihood of parasite infestation by following a few simple rules.

Wash your hands frequently and thoroughly with soap, especially following personal elimination, following raw food preparation, and following personal contact with other people. Especially avoid contact between your hands and your face.

Taking *citrus seed extract* (also known as grapefruit seed extract) on every day of your trip and for at least 3 days following your trip greatly reduces the risk of parasite infestation. Available in health food stores, citrus seed extract comes in 1 to 4 ounce dropper bottles and in tablets. (The extract tastes terrible!) Follow the directions on the label.

If you prefer a pharmaceutical remedy, purchase *Pepto-Bismol* (bismuth subsalicylate) tablets at any drugstore. The dose is 2 tablets 3 times per day on every day of your trip and for at least three days following your trip. Be prepared for a black tongue and black stool from this product. You also can take Pepto-Bismol to treat diarrhea. **Caution: Do not take Pepto-Bismol with aspirin without further study or consultation with a pharmacist or knowledgeable health-care provider. Do not give to children with flu or chicken pox — their use of salicylate-like compounds may increase the risk of Reye's Syndrome.** How well do citrus seed extract and Pepto-Bismol work? Trekking groups using either remedy report little or no travelers' diarrhea.

Don't eat raw or undercooked meat or fish. Many microorganisms live in raw meat, poultry, and fish. Many parasites survive searing, flash frying, or other quick cooking methods that leave the meat succulent, juicy, and rare. Most of them are killed by high heat or extended cooking. You don't need to order your meat burnt, but I would order at least medium to avoid parasites.

Don't eat sushi. Come on, you say, I've eaten sushi for years. Me, too. But it only takes 1 time with parasites to swear off sushi for a long, long time. I LOVE sushi. Still, eating sushi is a bit like Russian roulette. Eventually the bullet will be in the

PARASITES

chamber. So I no longer have sushi every week. Oh, you say you only have the cooked or vegetable sushi? Sorry, you are still at risk. The knife and the cutting board that touches the raw fish also touches YOUR California roll!

Do not eat raw shellfish.

In areas known for water contamination, you need to be especially careful to *avoid local water*. In water, parasites can survive simple chlorination. Drink only bottled, well purified, or recently boiled water. *Do not use ice cubes.* Do not use ice cubes in the hotel. Do not use ice cubes on the airline that is coming from or going to an area with water contamination — moving water to a plane does NOT eliminate the parasites. Travelers in Nepal recently were stricken with giardia — a particularly nasty single cell parasite — after they drank milk. The milk had been "thinned" with the local water — a common practice!

In areas with known water contamination, *eat no raw salad* — it would have been cleaned with contaminated water. *Eat cooked vegetables and cooked fruit.* If you eat raw fruit, only eat fruit that you peel yourself. If you must have raw vegetables or fruit, clean them thoroughly in a combination of bottled water and citrus seed extract.

Brush your teeth with bottled water.

Herbal Remedies for Parasites

Parasites have plagued humans for thousands and thousands of years, and people have found numerous botanical remedies. You can find herbal and food remedies in groceries, natural food stores, gardens, fields, and herb shops. Many are easy to use and extremely effective. Many work as well or better than many of the high priced drugs; many anti-parasite drugs ALSO work extremely well. In some situations, drugs are the best choice.

Most commercial herbal preparations for parasites contain a combination of herbs. Several of the herbs kill parasites, some may reduce cramping that may occur with parasite die-off, and others may help to move them out through the colon. Herbs you may find in parasite remedies include the following:

Black walnut hull	*Mugwort*
Cascara sagrada	*Pau d'arco*
Cat's claw	*Pink root*
Chaparro amargosa (NOT Chaparral)	*Quassia bark*
	Rhubarb
Clove	*Senna*
Garlic	*Thyme*
Goldenseal	*Wormwood*
Male fern	

Although no single herb (that I am aware of) will kill all parasites, I have seen great success with the combination of *wormwood, black walnut hull, cascara sagrada, and clove*. That is the combination I used! (See the beginning of the Parasites chapter.) Quassia bark or chaparro amargosa, a desert plant that also is known as *Castela emoryi*, are other great choices, especially if giardia is suspected.

To treat parasites, I would take a dose of the herbal combination every 20 minutes until symptoms shift (at least 3 times during the first 24 hours). Then, take 1 dose daily for the next 9 days. It is important to rest from the herbs for 7 days to allow any eggs to hatch. Then, resume the herbs for 10 more days. If symptoms do not shift or only partially improve, increase the frequency. If this treatment does not work, change your herbs and consider changing your anti-parasite strategy.

Anti-parasite herbs tend to be exceedingly bitter, and most people prefer tinctures or capsules. I recommend 1–2 droppersful of the tincture as a standard dose or 1–2 capsules. If the combination contains a laxative, it will send you to the bathroom with pretty loose stool. Keep drinking water and persevere.

Foods for Eliminating Parasites

Pumpkin seeds will reduce infestation. Available in grocery stores, natural food stores, and sometimes packaged as a snack food (check out Pumpkorn), eating at least ¹/2 cup of pumpkin seeds per day will reduce infestation. Worms don't like pumpkin seeds. While they are NOT a cure, they are useful in addition to other remedies. Choose raw seeds if possible — they may be more effective than roasted seeds.

Eating raw brown or white rice for breakfast is a traditional Tibetan and macrobiotic preventative and remedy for infestation. Carefully chew a quarter cup (1 handful) of raw rice before eating any other food. Chew as thoroughly as possible. Preferably, wait at least 3 hours before taking any additional food. Eat raw rice for 10 days, rest 5–7 days, and repeat for an additional 10 days. On days that you eat raw rice, an *herbal anti-parasite tea* is especially helpful. Good choices include *mugwort* (artemisia) or *fennel*. For severe infestation, fast on raw rice for 10 days and take anti-parasitic herbs.

Homeopathic Remedies for Parasites

You say that you treated for parasites but that you still have parasite symptoms? Homeopathic remedies for parasites may finish the job. A dose of homeopathic Giardia 6x, taken 3 times per day, may stop giardia related symptoms in less than 24 hours. Sometimes hard to find, homeopathic Giardia and other homeopathic remedies for parasites can be obtained from homeopaths, at some natural food stores, and on the Internet.

Summary of Parasite Remedies

Avoid parasites:

- Wash hands frequently.
- Take citrus seed extract daily.
- Don't eat raw or undercooked meat or fish.
- Eat cooked vegetables — no raw salad!
- Eat only cooked fruit or fruit you peel yourself.
- Drink only bottled or purified water. Chlorine is NOT enough!
- Don't use ice. Don't use ice. Don't use ice.
- Brush your teeth with bottled water.

Herbal remedies for parasites:

- Black walnut, clove, cascara sagrada, and wormwood, among others.

Foods for eliminating parasites:

- Pumpkin seeds.
- Raw rice.

Prescription drugs for eliminating parasites:

- Flagyl, among others.

PARASITES

STIFFNESS

In my thirties, I was privileged to fence for the Atlanta Fencers Club (AFC). Fencing is a sport that involves 5–10 minute bouts of intense activity followed by sedentary periods while one waits for the next bout. Between the beginning of competition at 8 a.m. and the end of competition at 8 p.m. (or even past midnight) a fencer might fence 30 bouts.

I remember one year when AFC competed at the Carolina Open, a two-day event featuring the strongest and largest field of fencers in the Southeast. We jammed five of us plus all our gear into a compact car and drove seven hours straight through to Chapel Hill, the home of the University of North Carolina. Safe at our destination, we unfolded and shook ourselves, trying to shake off our stiffness. We ate dinner, planning for the days ahead. On day one we would give our best for our team; on the second day we would compete in individual competition. Later, we would spend hours in the car driving home.

Oh, did we get stiff!

Stiffness occurs when we spend too long a period in a single position. It has happened to us all. You sit in a single position for hours on end. Four or 8 or maybe even 12 hours pass. You try to stand and your body seems permanently locked into position. Your joints seem stuck.

Stiffness also occurs when we do too much. Athletes become stiff when they do more than their accustomed training. They compete, rest, and stiffen up.

Travelers experience the double whammy of stiffness sufferers: They spend too long in a single position and then over-exert. Think of the times that you have walked and run for planes and trains while dragging heavy bags. Then, think of all the times you have sat in a car, on a bus, in a train, or on a plane, immobile for hours at a time after all that exertion, only to arrive at your destination and over-exert yourself again.

That time at the Carolina Open I was wide open for stiffness from both over-exertion and under-activity. On Saturday, AFC fenced team after team: Each of us fenced four bouts per team. Looking around the stadium, we saw what seemed to be innumerable teams that we had not yet fenced but would fence before the day ended. We fenced past midnight for a total of 16 hours of stop-and-go activity. Exhausted, we ate and fell into our beds.

The next morning, the alarm rang at 6 a.m. Four of us were in the room. All awakened at the alarm. None of us moved. I tried to move and could not! It seemed as though my joints had frozen. The alarm continued to ring. Someone called out, "Isn't anyone going to shut that thing off?" Apparently not. The alarm stopped on its own. We lay there, no one moving. Someone asked, "Aren't we fencing today?"

I did not know if I could fence. I did not know if I could get out of bed.

Eventually, we rose, one at a time, to the call of nature.

We dressed for day two.

We began the competition, keeping silent about our stiffness. I felt a bit embarrassed about feeling so stiff. "Getting old?" I wondered. I didn't want to show weakness, so I told no one.

Despite my stiffness I felt confident: I was highly seeded in the event and my first-round bouts were to be with less experienced fencers. I would need to win only three of the next five bouts to advance to the second round. As usual, I began my pre-competition warm-ups. Movement was difficult, and I decided that I would warm up in the first round.

In my first bout I marveled at my sluggishness and watched in amazement as a rank beginner shut me out. That's OK, I thought, I can drop one. I tried stretching before the next bout, running in place, and jumping up and down. For the second bout, I turned up the intensity level. I tried to be fast, I tried

STIFFNESS

to be devious, I tried to be clever. I kept fighting my body — and I lost. Two down, 3 to go.

Clearly, my warm-up was not enough.

I had about 20 minutes before my next bout. I began jogging around the perimeter of the stadium, moving from a jog to a run as soon as my body allowed. When would this clear? It seemed as though lactic acid ran through my veins, and I felt as though I were underwater. Every joint was stiff. All of my muscles ached. After about 15 minutes the stiffness and the aches began to ease. I ran until my next bout was called. Bout number 3. I needed to win.

With the warmth and the movement from my run, I felt looser, more flexible, and less tight. I focused on my opponent and won my bout. Now it was time to prepare for bout number 4. Typically, I would sit to conserve my energy while I mentally prepared. Not this time! There was no sense in conserving my energy if I were going to lose. I took off on another jog around the stadium and returned for my next bout. Sure, I was getting tired, but the stiffness was leaving. I won the next two bouts, easily. I began to feel like myself again.

[Epilogue: All of us made it to the semi-finals or the finals. I squeaked into the finals and came home with a medal, aching, exhausted, and very happy.]

What Causes Stiffness?

Western medicine tells us that over-exertion stiffness occurs when lactic acid accumulates in our tissues. Chinese medicine tells us that whole-body stiffness, either from over- or under-exertion, results from the accumulation of excess "wind-dampness." Athletes commonly explain mid-performance stiffness by saying they sat too long and got cold. Seniors struggle to stand and say that they sat still for too long. The West, the East, athletes, and seniors all speak of stiffness as resulting from a lack of movement. Let's call it stagnation.

Avoiding and Clearing Stiffness

Folk wisdom reminds us that a moving hinge never rusts. Stagnation is what allows rust (or lactic acid) to accumulate. *So keep moving!* Coaches recommend that athletes cool down and stretch following intense activity. That is great advice. Coaches recognize that intense activity results in our producing lactic acid and that moderate activity clears lactic acid. After running or fast walking to the plane, train, or bus, most of us plop down into the nearest chair. The result of our intense activity is lactic acid, which stagnates when we plop down. Don't plop! Instead, I recommend that you keep moving. *Walk. Stretch. Do simple calisthenics.*

"Keep moving!" also applies to under-exertion

STIFFNESS

problems of plane, train, bus, and car travel. Try to get up and walk or gently exercise every 1 or 2 hours. Yes, even when driving, you may wish to pull in to a rest area or a town. Five minutes of walking and stretching every hour will lengthen a car trip slightly but will greatly reduce or eliminate stiffness.

So you say that you are confined to your airline seat? There's turbulence or the person in the aisle seat is sleeping and walking around is impossible? You still can move and exercise many of your joints. Done systematically, you can reduce or even eliminate stiffness from extended sitting. These exercises also could be done at your desk or at a seated event such as a concert or lecture when you feel yourself becoming stiff.

Seated Flex and Rotate Exercises to Combat Stiffness and Increase Flexibility

Flex and rotate all of your joints at least 10 times each. Begin with your toes and work your way up the body.

■ *Toes:* Sit back in your seat. Flex, squeeze, and wiggle your toes. Rotate them clockwise, then counter-clockwise. Feel awkward? No worries, this will improve with time.

■ *Ankles:* Sit back in your seat. Lift your feet off the floor by extending your legs slightly. Flex your ankles by pointing your feet down and away from your body and then reverse the flex by pulling your feet up and towards your body. Rotate your feet clockwise and then counter-clockwise.

■ *Knees:* Sit back in your seat. Extend your legs by straightening them, then flex them by bending your legs at the knees. Rotate your lower legs clockwise, then counter-clockwise.

■ *Hips:* Sit forward in your seat so that your back no longer touches the back of the seat. Flex your hips by moving them as far as you can to the right, the left, the front and the back. (You CAN do this sitting!) If you can stand, place your feet together and circle your waist and hips clockwise and counter-clockwise. Spread your feet shoulder width apart and circle your waist and hips clockwise and counter-clockwise.

■ *Upper and Middle Back:* Sit forward in your seat. Flex your spine by slowly twisting your upper torso to the right and then to the left. Next, imagine that a flexible rubber hose stands up straight and in the center of your body. Rotate your upper body so that it moves clockwise around the hose, and then counter-clockwise. During the rotations your back will briefly touch the back of the seat, then your left side will move slightly to the left, then your chest and abdomen will move forward carrying you away from the back of the seat, then your right side will move slightly to the right. This will feel GREAT.

- *Shoulders:* Sit forward in your seat. Lift your shoulders up towards your ears as high as they will go and then drop them down towards your hips. Now, imagine you are a weight lifter and rotate your shoulders forward while your elbows come forward and then rotate your shoulders back behind you so that your elbows touch the back of the seat and your chest comes forward. Ahh. Next, perform "windshield washer arms." Bring your right arm in front of you with a bent elbow, vertical forearm and open palm facing to the left. Pivoting around your right elbow, press your right hand down towards your left hip and return your hand to an upright position. Do this on both the right and left sides.

- *Neck: Perform all neck exercises slowly and gently!* Sit forward in your seat. Drop your chin towards your chest, relax, and feel the stretch in your upper back. Slowly straighten your neck and move your head back as far as it will comfortably go. Relax and jut your jaw towards the ceiling. Gently, slowly, repeat. Next, turn your head as far as it comfortably will go, to the right. Gently return to center and repeat to the left side. Look as far to the left as you can. What about the rotations? Some people experience difficulties with neck rotations, so I have not included them. If they are part of your regular exercise program, by all means, do them!

- *Elbows:* Sit forward or back in your seat. Place

STIFFNESS

your elbows on your hips and your palms on your thighs. Pivoting at the elbow, raise your forearms off your thighs with your palms facing out, and gently return your forearms to your thighs. Next, keep your elbows on your hips and raise your forearms so that they are halfway between your legs and chest. Pivoting on your elbows, make circles in the air with your forearms. Reverse the circles.

■ *Wrists:* Place your elbows on your hips. Raise your forearms halfway between thigh and chest, with palms facing each other, fingers pointing up. Holding your forearms steady, press both palms together so that your fingers come close together. Then, pointing your fingers down, press the backs of your hands together. Relax and repeat. Then, still holding your forearms steady, make circles in the air with your hands. Reverse the circles.

■ *Hands:* Place your elbows on your hips. Raise your forearms halfway between thigh and chest, with palms facing each other. Holding your forearms steady, make tight fists and hold for a count of five, then open your hands as wide as you can and hold for a count of five.

Treating Stiffness

Taking a long, easy *walk* at the end of the day will help keep the kinks out. My personal favorite is to take a long *hot bath in Epsom salts.* I recommend that you add at least 1 cup of Epsom salts to a tub of water. Stir the salts into the bath to dissolve them and plan on soaking at least 10–15 minutes. This can be a life saver. If you wish to add essential oils to the bath, 10 drops of *lavender essential oil* is an excellent choice.

If you prefer showers, you might *try a contrast shower*. Stand under hot water, then switch to the coldest water you can stand, then switch to hot water. I recommend three to five full cycles. I did this following an intense 12-hour test for my black belt. It works!

An Eastern European coach taught me a sure-fire remedy for use when the next day's performance is critical. It is a harsh remedy, but I include it here because it is THE BEST remedy that I have used for severe over-exertion stiffness. It works better if you have a separate bathtub and shower. Fill the tub with cold water and add a large bag of ice. Get into the tub and stay there at least 1–2 minutes. (He said 5 minutes.) Get out and stand in a hot shower until you have warmed yourself. If you don't have a separate shower, roughly towel yourself, warming yourself with the friction. The coach said to repeat this process two more times. (I did not, and it still worked.) Do you need to do an ice bath? Only if contrast showers don't clear your stiffness and you MUST be at your peak the next day. I find it worth knowing.

STIFFNESS

Massage works! Massage, using deep and long strokes especially, helps to move lactic acid out and helps to relieve stagnation. Imagine that you accumulate puddles of lactic acid that cause stiffness and achiness and imagine that your kneading and stroking of the muscles helps to disperse those puddles. That is pretty close to what happens. Although having your own personal massage therapist certainly helps, you can gain many benefits from self-massage. I prefer to place most of my attention on the large muscles, such as the quadriceps muscles on the top of the thigh. Doing this in the hot Epsom salts bath makes it more beneficial.

Drink water. Drink 1 quart (32 ounces) or 1 liter (about 33 ounces) of water (not beer!) within a five-minute period. This signals the body to begin flushing itself and will send you repeatedly to urinate. Interestingly, you may urinate more than the amount that you drink! Continue drinking at least 8 ounces (1 cup) per hour. Drinking water in this manner will flush your system of accumulated lactic acid and toxins and will restore the water balance in your body.

You might want to try *apple cider vinegar*. Vinegar has an alkalizing effect on the body and helps to counteract the build-up of lactic acid. Try 1 tablespoon in a large glass of water. I like vinegar water just the way it is, but many people prefer to

STIFFNESS

add a teaspoon of honey. Either way, vinegar will help you to avoid stiffness. Take it at the beginning of a travel or a high activity day and again at day's end. This works for both over- and under-exertion stiffness.

Homeopathic Remedies

OK, so you prefer to just pop a pill. Be that way! Homeopathic *Arnica* is available in many health and natural foods stores, usually in tiny sugar pills. I recommend the lower potencies (6c to 30c) for dealing with stiffness. Take 1–3 at least 1 time and repeat up to every 15 minutes. I would take them prior to engaging in physical activity and before going to bed. Arnica also will help with recovery from aches and pains, bumps, and bruises. Be prepared for very rapid and sometimes dramatic results. See "Choosing Homeopathic Remedies," page 12.

If Arnica does not seem to help, especially if you sat for hours on end, if you endured extensive bumpy rides (off-road travel), or if your bruising occurred at a deep level, try homeopathic *Bellis perennis 30c* (English daisy). Although Arnica will work for almost everyone, Bellis can restore areas that Arnica cannot reach.

If your stiffness improves with movement and worsens with inactivity, try *Rhus toxicodendron 30c.*

Herbal and Food Remedies

An excellent tincture combination that is phenomenal for backaches and stiffness is *Back Support* from Rainforest Remedies — 1 dropperful 3 times per day.

For whole body stiffness that is due to cold (from long periods of sitting, especially in cold places), try multiple doses of *ginger*. Ginger tea, ginger tincture, ginger candy, ginger capsules — all will work. *Cayenne pepper* capsules also will warm and stimulate — take 2 capsules 1–3 times per day. Cayenne pads, salves, or oils effectively warm the skin and can relieve local pain — do NOT apply to sensitive tissues!

The Ayurvedic medical tradition suggests taking *turmeric* for stiffness — the recommended daily dose is 2 tablespoons. This may be taken daily in water or (more traditionally) in 1/2 cup of milk.

Umeboshi paste neutralizes lactic acid. Take 1/2 teaspoon of umeboshi plum or paste 1–3 times per day. This food remedy consists of a type of very sour plum that has been preserved in salt. Find it in your health food store.

Magnetic Therapy

You can use magnetic therapy to reduce or eliminate stiffness. A *therapeutic magnet*, applied directly to the site of pain, reduces pain in many people. If

STIFFNESS

the pain increases, flip the magnet over. Most people secure the magnet in place with tape or a Band-Aid. An individual therapeutic magnet will cost between $5 and $50. For whole body stiffness, a magnetic seat pad, mattress pad, or travel pad works very well for many people. The $100–400 price tag is WELL worth it. Smaller magnets are available in drug and health food stores. Magnetic pads are available on the Internet and through multi-level marketing. Some multi-level sellers will allow you to borrow a pad for the night so you can test the pad for yourself. Nikken, a multi-level company, sells excellent magnetic products.

Over-the-Counter Remedies

You say that showers, baths, herbs, and magnets are unavailable and you just want a drug? Sometimes you've got to do what you've got to do. Although these drugs will not eliminate the cause of the stiffness, they will relieve your discomfort. Most over-the-counter analgesic or anti-inflammatory drugs will help: *aspirin*, *ibuprofen* (Advil or Motrin), and *acetaminophen* (Tylenol).

My Choices

When I travel to the annual National Women in Martial Arts Federation conference, I ALWAYS bring a magnetic travel pad, Back Support by

Rainforest Remedies, and Arnica 30c. Does that make me a hypochondriac? Not at all! Only my roommate knows what I bring, and I don't have to be in pain. Although I am getting older, I am becoming craftier, and I experience very little stiffness.

Stiffness Summary of Remedies

Keep moving:
- Change your position.
- Walk.
- Stretch.
- Flex and rotate all joints.

Hydrotherapy:
- Epsom salts bath.
- Contrast shower (alternating hot and cold water).
- Ice bath followed by long warm shower.

Food, water, herbs, and supplements:
- Water.
- Apple cider vinegar.
- Arnica.
- Ginger or cayenne.
- Turmeric.
- Umeboshi plum.
- Back Support by Rainforest Remedies.

Therapeutic magnets:
- Individual magnets.
- Magnetic seat pads, mattress pads, or travel pads.

STIFFNESS

MAKING A TRAVEL KIT

As a child, first aid kits fascinated me. I've always liked the idea of being prepared. My father loved to fish, and he would take me with him to the local sporting goods store. I would run to the first aid kits and try to act like an adult shopper as I carefully opened each kit and considered the contents. Some had nothing more than Band-Aids, while others had smelling salts, aspirin, and special suction devices for snake bite. Really! The people who manufactured these kits seemed to think that the only thing that happened to people was that they would cut themselves, faint, get a headache, or get bitten by snakes.

I was indignant. I remember complaining to my parents that the kits were silly. Didn't anyone ever look inside these kits? My mother listened thoughtfully and then asked, "What items do you want in a kit?" I didn't know. That was the point of looking at all of those kits. I wanted to learn how to be prepared by seeing the items other people chose. She then asked, "What things have happened when you were outside or inside or playing or at school?"

That helped! Be prepared for what you have

experienced or seen. I knew what I had experienced. I had splinters — so I would include a needle, matches to sterilize the needle, and tweezers to pull out the splinter. My mom sometimes had an upset stomach, so I would include a stomach remedy for her. I also would include a pen-knife just in case someone couldn't breathe and needed a tracheotomy. (I had seen this on TV.) I also would include a set of directions to remind people what everything was for.

Now, with a few more years of experience, it is easier to think of what has happened and to anticipate what may happen on a trip. I am traveling all the time and constantly coping with life's challenges. I no longer limit my thinking to what might happen in the woods.

It would be easy to assemble a huge kit that contains remedies for hundreds of problems, but that would not be convenient. After all, who wants to travel with the equivalent of a small pharmacy? Now I ask what challenges I might expect to encounter and what multi-purpose remedies will be helpful.

Multi-Purpose Remedies

Multi-purpose remedies assist with a variety of health challenges, enabling us to carry less and do more. Many herbs are multi-purpose remedies and do far more than what a simple advertisement would suggest. (Why don't we hear more about the multiple uses of herbs or other remedies? Well, for one thing, companies make more money selling us many remedies rather than a single remedy. Also, marketing experts know that we are more likely to purchase when the message is simple.)

Multi-purpose remedies are listed throughout this book. Here they are again, listed in alphabetical order. For more information, consult the index and read the relevant section.

Herbs

■ *Cayenne pepper.* Warming. Treats muscle pain, bruises. Relieves sore throat and bronchitis. Use aggressively at the beginning of cold or flu to avoid the illness. Stimulates the heart, treats collapse, coma. Clears digestive congestion. Stops internal and external bleeding. Do NOT use internally when pregnant, when there are bladder problems, or for non-respiratory inflammation.

■ *Comfrey.* Number one remedy to stop bleeding, anywhere in the body. Number one remedy to accelerate all wound healing. Heals ulcers. Relieves dryness and relieves fatigue. Reduces inflammation and pain. But see "The Safe Use of Comfrey," page 40.

■ *Echinacea root.* Number one remedy for reducing viral and bacterial infection and fever and inflammation. Boosts immunity. Number one epidemic preventative. External antiseptic. Treats many poisons: internal and external remedy for snake bites. Assists with boils and many skin conditions, including gangrene and septic ulcers. Stimulates digestion. Detoxifying.

■ *Ginger*. Number one remedy for treating motion sickness and nausea. Treats indigestion, food poisoning, and stomach, abdominal, and menstrual cramps. Stimulates digestion, stops vomiting. Warming. Stops diarrhea from cold. Helps pain of arthritis, sore muscles. Use aggressively at the beginning of cold or flu to avoid the illness. Relieves colds. General anti-infective and epidemic preventative.

■ *Ginkgo*. Helps prevent and relieve altitude sickness. Also for mental sharpness and to improve circulation to the hands and feet.

■ *Pills Curing*. Chinese herbal combination remedy for indigestion, diarrhea, constipation, and stomach flu.

■ *Siberian ginseng*. Energy tonic, adrenal tonic. Stimulates immunity. Increases aerobic capacity.

Essential Oils

■ *Lavender essential oil*. Number one remedy for burns. Relaxant that relieves anxiety and depression. Calming. External remedy for pain, itching, and insect and spider bites. Apply directly to wounds to relieve pain, disinfect, reduce inflammation, accelerate healing, and reduce scarring. Eliminates lice, scabies, and other skin parasites. Apply to linen to eliminate bedbugs. Anti-viral: Steam inhalation (2–4 drops in 1 cup recently boiled water) for respiratory infections including colds, flu, bronchitis, and tuberculosis.

■ *Tea tree oil.* Anti-bacterial. Anti-viral. Anti-fungal. Steam inhalation (2–4 drops in 1 cup recently boiled water) to relieve colds, flu, bronchitis, and throat problems. One drop in 4 ounces of water used as a mouthwash, relieves toothache. Can be applied directly to the skin with or without diluting. Anti-infective for skin use.

■ *Thyme essential oil.* Number one remedy for all respiratory infections, including colds, flu, bronchitis, and pneumonia. Anti-bacterial. Anti-viral. Steam inhalation (2–4 drops in 1 cup recently boiled water) to relieve colds, flu, bronchitis, coughs, and throat problems. Anti-fungal. Anti-parasitic. Antidotes poison, including animal and insect bites. Major restorative: Clears fatigue, weakness, and nervous exhaustion. For internal use, place 1–2 drops with olive oil in a gelatin capsule, or stir 1–2 drops into a half teaspoon of honey and a quarter cup of water. One drop in 4 ounces of water used as a mouthwash relieves toothache. **Caution: Must be diluted for internal or external use.**

Homeopathics

- *Acidil or Nux vomica 30c.* Number one remedy for overindulgence in food or drink. Relieves hangovers, nausea, indigestion, sour stomach, diarrhea, and general digestive distress. See "Choosing Homeopathic Remedies," page 12.
- *Arnica 30c.* Number one remedy for accidents, trauma, swelling, and exhaustion.

Other

- *Charcoal.* Internal and external anti-poison. Treats indigestion.
- *Grapefruit seed extract.* Number one preventative for travelers' diarrhea. Clears yeast and mold.
- *Rescue Remedy.* Flower essence combination. Number one general remedy for emotional support.
- *Umeboshi plum paste.* Relieves indigestion, diarrhea, dysentery, stiffness, and crying.

Single-Purpose Remedies

Sometimes a single-purpose remedy is so outstanding that you will choose it in place of or in addition to a multi-purpose remedy. For example, when traveling in areas known for contaminated water supplies where travelers commonly develop diarrhea, I personally would bring the drug *Imodium.* It does one thing. It does that one thing extremely well. It stops diarrhea. Period.

You may wish to carry certain herbs, homeopathic preparations, or essential oils as single-purpose remedies. All of them will have multiple uses, but you may choose to focus on one.

Herbs

- *Astragalus root* tincture to boost immunity. Can be combined with echinacea.
- *Blackberry root bark* tincture to stop diarrhea.
- *Chaparro amargosa* or *quassia bark* for giardia and other parasites.
- *Mugwort (Artemisia annua)* for malaria.
- *Yunnan Paiyao* to stop bleeding.

Homeopathics

- *Apis 30c.* Number one remedy for bites and stings that burn and are red.
- *Arsenicum 30c.* Number one remedy for diarrhea accompanied by vomiting or for any suspected food poisoning.
- *Coca 30c.* Excellent homeopathic remedy for altitude sickness.
- *No Jet-Lag.* Number one combination remedy for jet lag and related travel problems.
- *Rhus toxicodendron 30c.* Number one preventative and treatment remedy for poison ivy and poison oak. Helpful for joint pain that is improved by motion and worsened by heat and humidity.

Assembling Your Travel Kit

The recommendations below are based upon creating a travel kit of reasonable size. Use the list as a start for developing your own kit. Many of the remedies are multi-purpose. If you commonly experience or anticipate a particular issue, I suggest that you review the relevant section in this book and tailor the kit to meet your needs.

Comprehensive Travel Kit

Blackberry root bark tincture

Ginger root tincture

Echinacea root tincture

Siberian ginseng root tincture

Lavender essential oil

Tea tree oil or thyme essential oil

Yunnan Paiyao

Rescue Remedy

Acidil or Nux vomica 30c

(Apis 30c — optional: include for hiking, trekking, swimming, and camping)

Arnica 30c

Arsenicum 30c

(Rhus toxicodendron 30c — optional: include for hiking, trekking, and camping)

Grapefruit seed extract

Charcoal

Vitamin C

Herbal salve containing goldenseal or other antibiotic herbs or pharmaceutical antibiotic ointment

Imodium

Earplugs

Sleep mask

Band-Aids — assorted sizes

Single edged razor blade or pen knife

Moleskin

Needle

Tweezers

1–2 empty dropper bottles: 1/2 or 1 ounce

Antibiotic skin cleanser that needs no water — 1 oz. size

Soap

Tissues in waterproof bag

1/2 inch wide first aid tape

Small lighter or waterproof matches

Small flashlight with batteries

List of all medications, herbs, homeopathics, and supplements you take

Water — small container

One copy of *The Healthy Traveler*

Here is a mini-kit that fits in your pocket:

Mini Travel Kit

Ginger tincture, Pills Curing, or Nux vomica 30c

Tea tree oil

Rescue Remedy

Band-Aids

List of all medications, herbs, homeopathics, and supplements you take

One copy of *The Healthy Traveler*

Foreign Phrases

English	German	French*
acupuncture	die Akupunktur	acuponcture
acupuncturist	der Akupunkteur	acuponcteur
ambulance	die Ambulanz	ambulance (f)
antibiotic	das Antibiotikum	antibiotique (m)
asthma	das Asthma	asthme
bandage	der Verband	bande (f) pansement (m)
bite	der Biss	piqure d'insecte (f) (insect bite)
bleeding	die Blutung	saignement (m)
breathing	atmen	respiration (f)
broken	gebrochen	cassé
Chinese	chinesisch	Chinois
chiropractor	der Chiropraktiker	chiropracteur (m)
constipation	die Verstopfung	constipation (f)
dentist	der Zahnarzt	dentiste (m)
diarrhea	der Durchfall	diarrhée (f)
drugstore	die Apotheke	pharmacie (f)
emergency	der Notfall	urgence épicerie (f)
essential oils	die Aetherische Öle	les huiles essentielles (f)
fever	das Fieber	fièvre (f)
flower essences	die Blütenessenzen	essences des fleurs (f)
food	die Nahrung	aliment (m)
grocery store	das Lebensmittelgeschaeft	supermarché (m) épicerie (f)

*The letters (m) and (f) denote gender (masculine and feminine).

Spanish	Italian	Portuguese
acupuntura	agopuntura	acupuntura
acupunturista	agopunturista	acupuntor
ambulancia	ambulanza	ambulância
antibiotico	antibiotico	antibiótico
asma	asma	asma
vendaje	fascia	atadura
picadura *(insect bite)*	insetto	picada
echar sangre	sanguinare	sangramento
respiracion	respirazione	respirar
fracturado *(bone)*	turato	cassado fraturado
Chino	Cinese	chinês *or* chinesa
quiropractico	chiropratico	quiroprático
estrenimiento	costipazione	constipação
dentista	dentista	dentista
diarrea	diarrea	diarréia
farmacia	farmacia	farmácia
emergencia	pronto soccorso emergenza	emergência
aceites esencials	olii essenziali	óleos essenciais
fiebre	febbre	febre
esencias florales	essenze floreali	essências de florais
comida	alimento	alimento
supermercado	supermercado	supermercado

English	German	French
herb	die Kräuter	fines herbes *(f)*
herb shop	das Reformhaus *or* das grüne Lädchen	herboristerie *(f)*
herbalist	der Kräuterhändler	herboriste
homeopath	der Homöopath	homéopathe
homeopathic	homöopathisch	homéopathique
homeopathy	die Homöopathie	homéopathie
massage	die Massage	massage *(m)*
medical doctor	der Arzt	docteur/médecin
medicine	die Medizin	médicament *(m)*
nurse	die Krankenschwester	infirmière *(f)*
osteopath	der Osteopath	ostéopathe
pain	der Schmerz	douleur *(f)*
restaurant	das Restaurant	restaurant *(m)*
sick	krank	malade
sting	stechen	piqure *(f)*
tea	der Tee	thé *(m)*
thirst	dürstig *(thirsty)*	soif
toilet	die Toilette	toilettes *(f)*
vomiting	erbrechen	vomissement *(m)*
water	das Wasser	eau *(f)*
good	gut	bon
bad	schlecht	mauvais
yes	ja	oui
no	nein	non

Spanish	Italian	Portuguese
hierba	erbe	erva
almacen de hierbas	erboristeria	loja de ervas
herborista	erborista	herborista
homeopath	omeopata	homeopata
homeopahische	omeopatico	homeopático
homeopathie	omeopatia	homeopatia
masaje	massaggio	massagem
doctor	medico	doutor
medicina	medicina	medicina
enfermera	infermiera	enfermeira
osteopata	osteopata	osteopático
dolor	dolore	dor
restaurante	ristorante	restaurante
enfermo	ammalato	doente
picadura	puntura	picada
te	té	chá
tener sed	sete	sede
retrete	gabinetto	higiênico
vomitos	vomito	vômito
agua	acqua	água
bueno	buono	bom
malo	difettoso	mau
si	si	sim
no	no	não

Terms

Essential Oils

Essential oils have been used for thousands of years and are the foundation for many perfumes and for aromatherapy. An essential oil is the distilled concentrate of a plant. Essential oils are the most highly concentrated of all herbal preparations. I think of 1 drop as being equivalent to 1 ounce of herb — essential oils are strong! One drop frequently is the dose, and that is enough. Treat all essential oils with respect; most must be diluted to prevent burning. (Lavender essential oil and tea tree oil are 2 common essential oils that you can safely use undiluted and that can be safely applied directly on the skin.) Essential oils are strongly anti-viral, antibiotic, and anti-fungal, making them potent alternatives to antibiotics. They are indispensable travel remedies due to their high concentration, consistent results, and easy portability. Practitioners are called aromatherapists.

Flower Essences

A flower essence is a low concentration tea (infusion) that has been further diluted in purified water (plus alcohol as a preservative). Flowers are usually used although bark or leaf may be used for some preparations. Flower essences are used to assist people with temporary or chronic emotional imbalances. The most common flower essence is Rescue Remedy, a combination of 5 flower essences. It is perfect in all high-stress situations. Most flower essences come in tiny dropper bottles. Flower essences provide rapid and gentle results without drug interactions or side effects.

Herbs

An herb is a plant, mineral, or animal that is used for healing. (Meat, bone meal, and gelatin all derive from animals.) Western herbology relies almost entirely on plants. Herbs are available in a wide variety of forms. All forms work. I personally rely on tinctures, which are extracts from herbs in alcohol and water, in glycerin, or in vinegar. Tinctures are easy to carry, easy to add to water to make tea, work very quickly, and stay fresh. Other forms include dried bulk herbs (the dried plant or plant part) which often is used for tea, tea bags, capsules (encapsulated ground bulk herbs), herbal oils (an extract from herbs in oil), salves (a herbal oil that has been solidified, usually with beeswax), and pills (ground and cooked herb molded into pill form). Practitioners are called herbalists or herbologists — you can find them by referral or by contacting an accrediting organization such as:

- American Herbalists Guild
  www.americanherbalist.com
- National Institute of Medical Herbalists
  www.btinternet.com/~nimh/
- European Herbal Practitioners Association
  (an umbrella organization for several accrediting
  organizations)
  www.users.globalnet.co.uk/~ehpa/about.htm

Homeopathic Remedies

A homeopathic remedy is an extremely low concentration preparation of a plant, mineral, or animal that is used for healing. The extremely low concentration allows the use of what otherwise would be poisonous, such as *Rhus toxicodendron* (poison ivy) to clear poison ivy rash and reduce arthritic pain. Most homeopathic remedies come in tiny pellets that dissolve under the tongue, in liquids in dropper bottles, or in a variety of skin lotions and gels. Correctly chosen, homeopathics are some of the most effective, least expensive, and easy to carry remedies. They are widely used in the United Kingdom, India, France, and other nations to treat a variety of conditions. Practitioners are called homeopaths and may be doctors of homeopathy or lay people — you can find outstanding practitioners in either group.

Resources

American Herbal Products Association. *Botanical Safety Handbook* (edited by Michael McGuffin, Christopher Hobbs, Roy Upton, Alicia Goldberg). Boca Raton, Florida: CRC Press, 1997.

Anderson, Bob. *Stretching.* Bolinas: Shelter Publications, 2000.

Auerbach, Paul S., Howard J. Donner, and Eric A. Weiss. *Field Guide to Wilderness Medicine.* St. Louis: Mosby, 1999.

Bergner, Paul. *The Healing Power of Ginseng and the Tonic Herbs.* Rocklin, California: Prima Publishing, 1996.

Boericke, William. *Homeopathic Materia Medica and Repertory.* Delhi: B. Jain (9th ed. 1927), reprinted 1996.

Bremness, Lesley. *Eyewitness Handbooks: Herbs.* New York: DK Publishing, 1994.

Balch, James F. and Phyllis A. *Prescription for Nutritional Healing.* Garden City Park, New York: Avery Publishing Group, 1997.

Chaltin, Luc. *Homeopathy for First Aid and Common Ailments.* Conyers, Georgia: The American Academy of Clinical Homeopathy, 1998.

Colbin, Annemarie. *Food and Healing.* New York: Ballantine, 1996.

D'Adamo, Peter J. with Catherine Whitney. *Eat Right for Your Type.* New York: G.P. Putnam's Sons, 1996.

Duke, James A. *The Green Pharmacy.* New York: St. Martin's Press, 1997.

Foster, Steven and James A. Duke, *A Field Guide to Medicinal Plants and Herbs of Eastern and Central North America.* Boston: Houghlin Mifflin Company, 2000.

Fratkin, Jake. *Chinese Herbal Patent Formulas: A Practical Guide.* Boulder, Colorado: Shyler Publications, 1997.

Gittleman, Ann Louise. *Your Body Knows Best*. New York: Pocket Books, 1996.

Graedon, Joe and Teresa. *The People's Pharmacy*. New York: St. Martin's Press, 1998.

Griggs, Barbara. *Green Pharmacy: The History and Evolution of Western Herbal Medicine*. Rochester, Vermont: Healing Arts Press, 1997.

Hass, Elson M. *Staying Healthy with Nutrition*. Berkeley, California: Celestial Arts, 1992.

Hass, Elson M. *Staying Healthy with the Seasons*. Berkeley, California: Celestial Arts, 1981.

Holmes, Peter. *The Energetics of Western Herbs, Vols. I and II*. Boulder, Colorado: Snow Lotus Press, 1997 (Vol. 1) and 1999 (Vol. 2).

Jarvis, D.C. *Folk Medicine*. New York: Fawcett Crest, 1958.

Kaminski, Patricia and Richard Katz. *Flower Essence Repertory*. Nevada City, California: Flower Essence Society, 1996.

Kaptchuk, Ted J. *The Web That Has No Weaver: Understanding Chinese Medicine*. Chicago, Illinois: Contemporary Books, 2000.

Kushi, Michio. *Macrobiotic Home Remedies*. Tokyo: Japan Publications, 1989.

Maciocia, Giovanni. *The Foundations of Chinese Medicine: A Comprehensive Text for Acupuncturists and Herbalists*. Edinburgh: Churchill Livingstone, 1998.

Maciocia, Giovanni. *The Practice of Chinese Medicine: The Treatment of Diseases with Acupuncture and Chinese Herbs*. Edinburgh: Churchill Livingstone, 1998.

Moore, Michael. *Medicinal Plants of the Desert and Canyon West*. Santa Fe, New Mexico: Museum of New Mexico Press, 1990.

Northrup, Christiane. *The Wisdom of Menopause*. New York: Bantam Books, 2001.

Northrup, Christiane. *Women's Bodies, Women's Wisdom*. New York: Bantam Books, 1998.

Pitchford, Paul. *Healing with Whole Foods: Oriental Traditions and Modern Nutrition.* Berkeley, California: North Atlantic Books, 1993.

Price, Weston. *Nutrition & Physical Degeneration.* New Canaan, Connecticut: Keats, 1989.

Reid, Daniel R. *The Tao of Health, Sex, & Longevity.* New York: Fireside, 1989.

Ross, Julia. *The Diet Cure.* New York: Viking, 1999.

Scheffer, Mechthild. *Mastering Bach Flower Therapies: A Guide to Diagnosis and Treatment.* Rochester, Vermont: Healing Arts Press, 1996.

Scheffer, Mechthild. *Bach Flower Therapy: Theory and Practice.* Rochester, Vermont: Healing Arts Press, 1988.

Tierra, Leslie. *The Herbs of Life: Health & Healing Using Western & Chinese Techniques.* California: Crossing Press, 1992.

Tierra, Michael. *The Way of Herbs.* New York: Pocket Books, 1990.

Tierra, Michael and Leslie. *Chinese Traditional Herbal Medicine, Vols. 1 and 2.* Twin Lakes, Wisconsin: Lotus Press, 1998.

Valnet, Jean. *The Practice of Aromatherapy: A Classic Compendium of Plant Medicines & Their Healing Properties* (edited by Robert Tisserand). Rochester, Vermont: Healing Arts Press, 1990.

Weil, Andrew. *Eating Well for Optimum Health.* New York: Quill, 2001.

Williams, Roger. *Nutrition Against Disease.* New York: Bantam, 1973.

Worwood, Valerie Ann. *The Complete Book of Essential Oils & Aromatherapy.* Novato, California: New World Library, 1991.

Index

About the Author

Susan W. Kramer was born in Brooklyn, New York and grew up in Perth Amboy, New Jersey, where she spent much of her time outdoors, active in sports and fascinated by the plants she discovered while tramping through the woods behind her home. After completing high school, she attended New College in Sarasota, Florida and Marlboro College in Marlboro, Vermont, graduating from New College in 1975 with a degree in economics and music. She earned an M.A. in economics and demography in 1977 and a Ph.D. in economics in 1978, both from Duke University, and taught economics at the College of William and Mary and George Washington University. Kramer took leave from academia in 1980, working as an economist first for the Federal Reserve Board of Governors and then for the U.S. House of Representatives. She returned to the College of William and Mary to study law, earning her J.D. in 1986, and practiced law for ten years, specializing in bankruptcy litigation. A longtime competitive athlete, Kramer has earned a second degree black belt in Bu Kyoku Ryu Karate and is a certified instructor of Tai Chi and a championship fencer. She served on the United States Fencing Association Board of Directors from 1986–1995.

Her lifelong interests in health and plants eventually led to advanced studies at the East West School for Herbology in Santa Cruz, California. She became accredited as a professional member of the American Herbalists Guild and a Reiki Master in 1998. Kramer is a member of the National Women in Martial Arts Federation and the Complementary and Alternative Medical Association (CAMA). She lives in Atlanta, Georgia, where she maintains a practice as a therapeutic herbalist. She also is president and founder of EarthWays Herbal Products, manufacturer of premium products for the active individual (www.earthways.com).